# Women Prisoners and Health Justice

This book is dedicated to women prisoners around the world.

# Women Prisoners and Health Justice

## PERSPECTIVES, ISSUES AND ADVOCACY FOR AN INTERNATIONAL HIDDEN POPULATION

Edited by

**DIANE C HATTON** RN DNSc

*Professor*
*School of Nursing*
*San Diego State University*
*San Diego, CA*

and

**ANASTASIA A FISHER** RN DNSc

*Associate Professor*
*School of Nursing*
*San Francisco State University*
*San Francisco, CA*

Foreword by

**ANDREW COYLE**

*Professor of Prison Studies*
*School of Law*
*King's College*
*University of London*

Radcliffe Publishing
Oxford • New York

**Radcliffe Publishing Ltd**
18 Marcham Road
Abingdon
Oxon OX14 1AA
United Kingdom

**www.radcliffe-oxford.com**
Electronic catalogue and worldwide online ordering facility.

British Library Cataloguing in Publication Data
A catalogue record for this book is available from the British Library.

ISBN-13: 978 184619 242 5

The paper used for the text pages of this book is FSC certified. FSC (The Forest Stewardship Council) is an international network to promote responsible management of the world's forests.

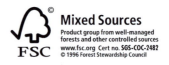

**Mixed Sources**
Product group from well-managed forests and other controlled sources
www.fsc.org Cert no. SGS-COC-2482
© 1996 Forest Stewardship Council

Typeset by Pindar NZ, Auckland, New Zealand
Printed and bound by TJI Digital, Padstow, Cornwall, UK

# Contents

# Foreword

The proportion of women in prison systems throughout the world varies between 2% and 9%, with only 12 jurisdictions having a higher proportion.[1] These figures do not mean that the total number of women in prison is small. Indeed, in many jurisdictions recent increases in the number of women in prison has exceeded the increase in male prisoners. It is estimated that there are over half a million women and children in prison, either sentenced or awaiting trial. Of these, one-third is in the US.

One consequence of the proportional imbalance of the sexes is that prisons and prison systems tend to be organized to meet the needs and requirements of male prisoners. This applies to architecture, to security and to all other facilities. There is a recurring tendency that any special provision for women prisoners will be something that is added on to the standard provision for men. This is despite the fact that the profile of women prisoners is very different from that of male prisoners, and particular attention should be given to their special needs.

Most women will have been imprisoned for non-violent property offenses. If their crime has been a violent one, the victim is likely to have been someone close to them. Many women prisoners will have suffered frequent physical or sexual abuse. They will often have a variety of untreated health problems. In addition, the consequences of imprisonment and its effect on their lives may be very different for women. A large number will be single parents, often with dependent children. When a man is sent to prison, his partner may well do all in her power to keep the family together. When a woman goes to prison, there is less likelihood that her partner will manage to do the same.

In a number of countries tough anti-drug legislation has had a significant effect on the numbers of women in prison. Another feature of this and similar changes has been an increase in the proportion of foreign national prisoners who now form a large percentage of women prisoners in some countries. All of these factors mean that prison authorities need to pay special attention to the way women prisoners are treated and the facilities that are provided for them.

This is especially so in terms of their health needs.

The health profile of prisoners as a whole is poor. This is not surprising, given the fact that in most jurisdictions prisoners are drawn largely from marginalized groups. Many will have untreated health conditions. A high proportion of them will be addicted to one or more drugs of abuse, with the added possibility that they may suffer from infectious hepatitis, tuberculosis or HIV. The incidence of mental health problems among prisoners is very high. If that is their condition when they enter prison, the environment in which they then live is likely to exacerbate their problems. In many instances living conditions may be badly overcrowded, sanitary arrangements may be poor, diet will be inadequate, there will be limited access to fresh air and exercise, and health provision will be unsatisfactory. For women in prison, many of these problems will be writ even larger.

This book, edited by Diane Hatton and Anastasia Fisher, fills a major gap in the literature on two counts: it is about women prisoners, and it is about their entitlement to proper health care. The editors have gathered a knowledgeable and experienced group of experts from around the world to contribute chapters on key issues on this topic. This volume is likely to become a classic reference text.

This book should be read by all those who are in any way involved in the imprisonment of women. But it is not only a book for practitioners, academics and prison policy makers. It also needs to be read by those involved in the world of health policy and health delivery and its lessons taken on board by them. The women who are described in this volume are a problematic group. Their health problems are complex and often not easily resolved. They may not always be grateful for help when it is offered. It is too easy for health professionals to ignore their problems, to put them into a category marked "too difficult." All health professionals should bear in mind the Oath of Athens passed in 1979 by the International Council of Prison Medical Services which pledged "in keeping with the spirit of the Oath of Hippocrates . . . we shall endeavor to provide the best possible health care for those who are incarcerated in prisons for whatever reasons, without prejudice and within our respective professional ethics. We recognize the right of the incarcerated individuals to receive the best possible health care."[2]

That commitment applies particularly to women who are in prison. This book serves to reinforce that pledge.

Andrew Coyle
Professor of Prison Studies
School of Law
King's College
University of London
*June 2009*

## REFERENCES

1 Walmsley R. *World Female Imprisonment List.* London: International Centre for Prison Studies; 2006.

2 Coyle A. *A Human Rights Approach to Prison Management.* London: International Centre for Prison Studies; 2002. p. 57. Available at: www.kcl.ac.uk/depsta/law/research/icps/downloads/human_rights_prison_management.pdf (accessed February 28, 2009).

# Preface

The past three decades have witnessed an unprecedented increase in the world-wide prison population that includes a burgeoning number of women. The US leads this trend with 25% of the world's prisoners, in spite of having only 5% of the world's population.[1] The US confines more than one in every 100 adults in a jail or prison[2] and although men are more likely to be incarcerated, the number of women prisoners has increased at a faster pace. In 2008, African-American women from age 35 to 39 reached the 1-in-100 mark.[2] The US patterns of incarceration, its disproportionately high convictions of the poor and racial/ethnic minorities, as well as its deteriorating prison conditions are found in other countries, including Canada, Australia, and the UK.[3]

Incarceration severely affects the health and well-being of women, and disproportionately impacts women of color who are incarcerated at substantially higher rates than their white counterparts.[4] When removed from their communities, incarcerated women are placed in jails and prisons where infectious and chronic diseases are frequently prevalent, and medical neglect exists in spite of the national and international documents that clearly define standards for health care. Eventually most women prisoners return to communities where they encounter difficulty accessing needed services, especially substance abuse and other mental health treatment. They also find limited opportunities for job training and employment, lack of adequate housing, and other circumstances that impede successful reentry and put them at substantial risk for recidivism.[5]

The scope of this international problem remains largely hidden from health professionals and policy makers. Although the majority of women prisoners are convicted of non-violent, drug-related crimes, the political discourse about this enormous increase in women's imprisonment often centers on public safety, and health is given little acknowledgement by politicians advancing their careers with tough-on-crime approaches.[6] This book analyzes how incarceration severely limits women's opportunities, damaging their health and that of their families and communities. The book also examines how imprisonment further complicates the health disparities women prisoners experience as a consequence of gender, race, and class, for typically they bear the burden of being poor, being female, being women of color, and having a history of a criminal conviction.[7] They commonly suffer multiple, persistent physical, mental, and social health problems.[4,8-13] Their pregnancy rates are higher than their cohorts in the general population and they often report histories of violence as children and as adults.[14,15] Compared with male prisoners, they are more likely to have been homeless, report drug charges at arrest, and be parents.[16] Research also indicates that during the first 12 months after release from prison, women's risk for suicide is higher than the general population and higher than recently released men.[17]

However, we have not organized this book around specific diseases or health problems as the reader can find these comprehensive accounts in the literature. We have taken a different approach by focusing on perspectives for examining health among women prisoners, including human rights and social capital. We consider specific circumstances related to their health and health care access, such as race, gender, class, and prison environments. We emphasize strategies for moving from knowledge to action that address health promotion, standards, codes of ethics, advocacy, and education.

## AIM OF THE BOOK

The aim of this edited book is to address the gap in knowledge about the health of women prisoners and it represents the outcome of a meeting organized by the editors and supported by the Rockefeller Foundation at their Study and Conference Center in Bellagio, Italy. During that meeting, our group discussed the ideas in this book and represented various viewpoints as advocates, criminologists, feminists, former prisoners, nurses, physicians, public health professionals, social workers, and sociologists. We began this effort with four countries – Australia, Canada, the UK and the US – because we speak a common language and our countries have similar legal traditions. We hope that future work will bring additional countries and perspectives to this discourse as the imprisonment of women has become a transnational, global phenomenon.[18]

## OVERVIEW OF THE BOOK

In this book we use the term "health" broadly, as does the World Health Organization (WHO), to include "physical, mental, and social well being and not merely the absence of disease or infirmity."[19] We also address women prisoners in a broad manner by considering not only those incarcerated but also those with a history of incarceration, such as women attempting to reenter the community after release from prison.

In Chapter 1, Anne Davis reviews the ethical and legal principle of justice, the conceptual frame for human rights. She explores the philosophical and historical support for human rights and considers the interaction between human rights and health. Davis asks health professionals and others aware of the socio-economic and political human rights issues surrounding the increased imprisonment of women to consider what model of justice benefits society and individuals. The values of justice and rights for all humans are foundational to this book's assumptions about what constitutes health problems for women prisoners and what actions to take in response.

In Chapter 2, Virginia Olesen situates the individual woman prisoner in a social context that allows us to think about how women secure benefits by virtue of their membership in social networks and other social structures. She explores how these networks assist or hinder women in accessing resources – both inside and outside prison. When thinking about reentry, she proposes exploration of those networks that will broaden the opportunities for successful reintegration to communities.

In Chapter 3, Beth Richie's seminal research article describes the challenges that incarcerated women face as they return to their communities from jail or prison. Richie's chapter provides thick description of social networks and structures that are critical for women, their children, and other family members. She points to the urgent need for social reform and argues that the challenges women face must be met by a more thoughtful criminal justice policy that requires reinvestment in low-income communities to reduce recidivism.

In Chapter 4, Judy Parker, Debbie Kilroy and Jonathan Hirst examine patterns of women's incarceration in Australia and focus particular attention on forensic mental health services as well as Aboriginal and Torres Strait Islander women within the criminal justice system. They demonstrate the health difficulties experienced and argue for a shift from prison-based to community-based care with provision of adequate social and health services. They discuss the mounting evidence that the prison environment exacerbates disadvantage and discrimination. They recommend strategies for community-based programs aimed at healing the wounds suffered by women who have been victims of an uncaring society.

In Chapter 5, Paul Godin and Kathleen Kendall also analyze the harmful effects of incarceration, focusing on the history of British women's prisons and paying particular attention to mental health. They argue that programs for women prisoners often focus on the mental pathology of individual women rather than on the numerous social processes that contribute to incarceration in the first place, such as social marginalization, policing, and sentencing practices. They support the implementation of gender-responsive programs for women prisoners.

In Chapter 6, Nancy Stoller's commentary explores ways that gender is managed through prison policies and practices. Considering racism and ethnicity, as well as gender, she examines how women's prison experiences cannot be understood through a lens that focuses primarily on men. Stoller describes how women prisoners who become ill or suffer unintended or intended trauma are already in a hostile environment where their identities, former lives, families, affectional ties, and self-agency are under attack. She argues that the intricate systems of racism and sexism present barriers to the delivery of jail and prison health care, and she discusses the discriminatory practices former prisoners encounter upon release.

In Chapter 7, Karlene Faith's commentary argues that prisons are antithetical to women's health. She presents data from interviews conducted with women prisoners in the US and Canada that illustrate the damaging effects of incarceration on health. She advocates a transformative model of justice that challenges a need for prisons in a civilized society. Like Anne Davis (Chapter 1), she acknowledges the physical, emotional, and mental harm to women prisoners as a human rights abuse. She proposes the ideals of transformative justice as a new way to think about the kind of society we want to inhabit.

In Chapter 8, Alex Gatherer, Lars Møller and Paul Hayton take a public health point of view and argue that one of the most urgent tasks of prisons is to improve the health, resilience, and well-being of all those in compulsory detention, especially women. They describe how this is in the women's best interests, and the interests of their families and others. They emphasize that the health of women prisoners is important to public health as a whole. Their chapter discusses the WHO Health in Prisons Project (HIPP) that was launched in 1995 in eight European countries. HIPP offers a model for the development of collaborative, multinational, and multidisciplinary relationships that address the challenges of prison health care.

In Chapter 9, Nancy Stoller and Alex Gatherer examine accreditation, standards, monitoring, professionalization, and community-based care provision as means of improving prison health care. They offer comparisons between the US and English systems that highlight the approaches taken in the two countries in prison health care and community-based care. The differences between the US and England demonstrate the significance of having one national health care system to provide a community standard of care inside prisons instead of a fragmented collection of services.

In Chapter 10, Janet Storch and Cindy Peternelj-Taylor borrow extensively from the Canadian Nurses Association (CNA) Code of Ethics for Registered Nurses (2008) to illustrate how codes can guide health providers' actions in practice. The chapter includes discussion of the dual responsibilities – control and care – health care professionals encounter in prisons. While recognizing prisons as unhealthy and detrimental places for all people, these authors argue that health professionals can do a great deal to offer respectful health-promoting care, to protect prisoners from research abuse, and to advocate for alternatives to imprisonment.

In Chapter 11, Donna Willmott builds on the ethical obligation for advocacy by exploring specific ways that health professionals may fulfill this obligation. She describes advocating for individual patient-prisoners, supporting the efforts of prisoners to advocate for themselves, and working with community-based organizations to ensure the rights and dignity of patient-prisoners through public education and policy change. Using examples of organizations in Australia, Canada, and the US, she demonstrates how collaboration between health providers, prisoners' rights advocates, prisoners and former prisoners can encourage policy change to lessen the negative impact of incarceration on individuals, families, and communities.

In Chapter 12, Judy Parker, Lisa Reynolds and Donna Willmott bring together many issues addressed in previous chapters and focus on the educational needs of professionals, policy makers, community workers, and members of the public concerned about the health status of incarcerated women. They argue that education can play a crucial role in shifting attitudes and values, and support curricula that broaden individuals' horizons and challenge stereotypical and negative ways of thinking about women in prison. They also recognize the importance of examining the socio-political and structural reasons that lie behind incarceration. They offer an emancipatory approach to curriculum development as a tool to improve the health and well-being of incarcerated women.

In Chapter 13, Anastasia Fisher, Diane Hatton and Jane Dorotik summarize the major points of the book and make recommendations for action. The latter include using jails and prisons sparingly, especially for non-violent offenses; replacing incarceration with community alternatives such as drug, mental health, and homeless courts; improving prison health care and programs; and supporting the conduct of ethical research with prisoners. Using California as an example, the chapter summarizes the problems of delivering health care when there is mass incarceration. The chapter concludes by arguing that societies have a choice: they can continue to punish mass numbers of individuals or reinvest in their communities and their children. This reinvestment includes tackling the problems of inequity, discrimination, and the paralyzing effects of poverty. Only then can health justice be achieved.

## SUMMARY

Imprisonment impacts women's physical, mental, and social health. Taking the perspective of women as creators of social capital, this book demonstrates how imprisonment further complicates the health disparities women prisoners already experience as a consequence of gender, race, and class. It also considers the collateral damage to families and communities as a consequence of women's imprisonment.[1,20] Estimates suggest, for example, that almost 70% of the women prisoners in the US are mothers. When they are incarcerated, their children are left behind with little protection or hope; these children are often forced into foster care and become vulnerable to the psychosocial problems that entails.[20]

This book offers different views on whether prison health care can be improved. Some say that prisons can and should be health-promoting settings; others suggest this is not possible. Our intention is to capture these various perspectives and acknowledge their tension. In spite of their differences, the contributors to this volume come from a human rights perspective, acknowledging that women have a right to health care, both in and out of prison. Thus, this collection of essays represents an effort to address and advocate for the health of women prisoners from a health justice perspective, which the editors understand as the fair and equal distribution of health resources in communities as well as in prisons. We use the term here to capture the idea that for health to be a possibility, inequities, discrimination, and the paralyzing effects of poverty must be addressed by societies around the world.

The physical, mental, and social conditions experienced by women prisoners, their minor children, their families, and their communities have not been adequately acknowledged or addressed by society as a whole or by those segments of society that could make a difference in their lives. Over our careers we have worked with persons who have mental illnesses, substance use disorders, and histories of homelessness. We have witnessed a shift in the location of these populations from traditional settings such as shelters, community health clinics, and psychiatric hospitals, to jails and prisons. In our communities, the local jails have now become the largest providers of mental health services. The health care system in our overcrowded California prisons has been placed under a federal receiver because its inadequate medical care violated the US Constitution's Eighth Amendment that forbids cruel and unusual punishment of incarcerated persons.[21]

We have presented this topic to medical residents, students in public health, nursing, social science, and liberal arts, custody staff, as well as international, national, regional, and local health professional groups. These presentations have illuminated the need for increased awareness about the global scope of the problems facing women prisoners and the health professionals responsible for their care. We hope this work will generate an interest among physicians, nurses, social workers, public health workers, health law professionals, policy makers, and other interested advocates to develop and implement strategies that will reduce avoidable and unfair differences in the health status of women prisoners.

Diane C Hatton
Anastasia A Fisher
*June 2009*

## REFERENCES

1 Drucker EM. Incarcerated people. In: Levy BS, Sidel VW, editors. *Social Injustice and Public Health.* Oxford: Oxford University Press; 2006. pp. 161–75.
2 PEW Center on the States. *One in 100: behind bars in America 2008.* Washington, DC: The PEW Charitable Trusts. Available at: www.pewcenteronthestates.org/uploadedFiles /One%20in%20100.pdf (accessed May 24, 2009).
3 Wood PJ. The rise of the prison industrial complex in the United States. In: Coyle A, Campbell A, Neufeld R, editors. *Capitalist Punishment: prison privatization and human rights.* Atlanta, GA: Clarity Press; 2003. pp. 16–29.
4 Braithwaite RL, Treadwell HM, Arriola KR. Health disparities and incarcerated women: a population ignored. *Am J Public Health.* 2005; **95**(10): 1679–81.
5 Freudenberg N, Daniels J, Crum M, *et al.* Coming home from jail: the social and health consequences of community reentry for women, male adolescents, and their families and communities. *Am J Public Health.* 2005; **95**(10): 1725–36.
6 Walmsley R. Prison planet. *Foreign Policy.* 2007; **160**(May/Jun): 30–1.
7 Freudenberg N. Adverse effects of US jail and prison policies on the health and well-being of women of color. *Am J Public Health.* 2002; **92**(12): 1895–9.
8 Stoller N. *Improving Access to Health Care for California's Women Prisoners.* Berkeley, CA: California Policy Research Center, University of California; 2001. Available at: http://cpac.berkeley.edu/documents/stollerpaper.pdf (accessed May 24, 2009).
9 Hatton DC, Kleffel D, Fisher AA. Prisoners' perspectives of health problems and healthcare in a US women's jail. *Women and Health.* 2006; **44**(1): 119–36.
10 National Commission on Correctional Health Care. *The Health Status of Soon-To-Be-Released Inmates: a report to congress.* Available at: www.ncchc.org/pubs/pubs_stbr. html (accessed November 5, 2008).
11 Federal Bureau of Prisons. *Management of Methicillin-Resistant Staphylococcus Aureus (MRSA) Infections.* Washington, DC: Department of Justice; 2005. Available at: www. bop.gov/news/PDFs/mrsa.pdf (accessed May 24, 2009).
12 Willmott D, van Olphen J. Challenging the health impacts of incarceration: the role for community health workers. *Californian J Health Promot.* 2005; **3**(2): 38–48. Available at: www.csuchico.edu/cjhp/3/2/38-48-willmott.pdf (accessed November 5, 2008).
13 Braithwaite RL, Arriola KJ, Newkirk C. *Health Issues Among Incarcerated Women.* New Brunswick, NJ: Rutgers University Press; 2006.
14 Fogel CI, Belyea M. Psychological risk factors in pregnant inmates. A challenge for nursing. *MCN Am J Matern Child Nurs.* 2001; **26**(1): 10–16.
15 Richie BE, Freudenberg N, Page J. Reintegrating women leaving jail into urban

communities: a description of a model program. *J Urban Health*. 2001; **78**(2): 290–303.

16 Freudenberg N, Moseley J, Labriola M, *et al*. Comparison of health and social characteristics of people leaving New York City jails by age, gender, and race/ethnicity: implications for public health interventions. *Public Health Rep*. 2007; **122**(6): 733–43.

17 Pratt D, Piper M, Appleby L, *et al*. Suicide in recently released prisoners: a population-based cohort study. *Lancet*. 2006; **368**(9530): 119–23.

18 Sudbury J, editor. *Global Lockdown: race, gender, and the prison-industrial complex*. New York, NY: Routledge; 2005.

19 World Health Organization. *WHO Definition of Health*. 1948. Available at: www.who. int/about/definition/en/print.html (accessed November 5, 2008).

20 Golden R. *War on the Family: mothers in prison and the families they leave behind*. New York, NY: Routledge; 2005.

21 California Prison Health Care Services. *California Prison Health Care Receivership Corp. About us*. 2008. Available at: www.cphcs.ca.gov/about.aspx (accessed November 5, 2008).

# About the Editors

**ANASTASIA FISHER**

Anastasia Fisher's early career experiences as a psychiatric nurse working with persons who live with serious mental illnesses together with her doctoral education at the University of California, San Francisco, where she was privileged to meet and study ethics with Dr. Anne Davis, were influential in shaping her interest in the ethical foundations of psychiatric nursing practice and human rights. Much of her career has focused on the education of nurses and others who work with vulnerable populations in forensic psychiatric and jail settings. She continues this work as an Associate Professor in the School of Nursing at San Francisco State University and through her current community-based participatory research program with Dr. Diane Hatton which focuses on health care access and health care justice for incarcerated women.

**DIANE HATTON**

Diane Hatton's work has focused on public health nursing and the care of vulnerable populations, especially women with histories of homelessness and imprisonment. Dr. Anne Davis influenced her interest in ethics when she was a doctoral student at the University of California, San Francisco. Her current research with colleague Dr. Anastasia Fisher builds on this ethics background and uses community-based participatory methods to consider the health and human rights of women prisoners. She is a Professor at San Diego State University where she also serves as the Associate Director for Research in the School of Nursing. She has chaired the Committee on Women's Rights of the American Public Health Association. Dr. Hatton and Dr. Fisher received an award from the Rockefeller Foundation that supported the initial meeting of this volume's contributors at their Study and Conference Center in Bellagio, Italy.

# List of Contributors

**ANNE DAVIS**

During 34 years at the University of California, San Francisco, Anne Davis established the nursing ethics program, served as a member of the Clinical Ethics Committee and the Research Ethics Committee, developed the ethics committee at Hospice by the Bay, chaired the California Nurses' Association and American Nurses' Association Ethics Committees and worked with graduate students on their research. She has visited 120 countries and worked in the Middle East, Europe, Africa, India, and China. For six years she worked at Nagano College of Nursing, Japan. Her major research interests are end-of-life ethics and international nursing ethics.

**JANE DOROTIK**

Jane Dorotik is incarcerated at the California Institute for Women (CIW). She works tirelessly to demand human rights for women who are imprisoned and to raise public consciousness about the struggles that women encounter on a daily basis while they are incarcerated. Jane also writes on the conditions of confinement and the abolition of prisons.

**KARLENE FAITH**

A native of Saskatchewan, Karlene Faith's PhD is from the History of Consciousness program at the University of California, Santa Cruz. She co-founded the Santa Cruz Women's Prison Project, an accredited university program in 1972, and Music Inside/Out in 1976, taking concerts to women's prisons. She returned to Canada in 1982, and is now Professor Emerita at Simon Fraser University in British Columbia, where she has been associated with the School of Criminology; Women's Studies; Centre for Distance Education; Secwepemc First Nations University; Institute for the Humanities; and Centre for Restorative Justice. She co-founded the Feminist Institute for the Study of Law and Society and SIS (Strength in Sisterhood), a national support and advocacy network of current or former prisoners. A long-time human rights activist, her publications include *13 Women: parables from prison* (with Anne Near) (Douglas & McIntyre; 2006), *The Long Prison Journey of Leslie Van Houten* (Northeastern University Press; 2001), and *Unruly Women: the politics of confinement and resistance* (Press Gang Publishers; 1993).

## ALEX GATHERER

Alex Gatherer's main career as a public health physician was in Oxford, UK where he was deeply involved in issues relating to the management and medical staffing of a well-known teaching hospital and health service. He was invited in 1994 to be a temporary adviser to a new World Health Organization (Europe) network of countries committed to exchanging experiences and ideas on how to improve health care in prisons throughout Europe. He has remained as adviser since then and works closely with the manager of what has become known as the WHO Health in Prisons Project, Dr. Lars Møller, based in the WHO Regional Office for Europe, Copenhagen, Denmark.

## PAUL GODIN

Paul Godin is Senior Lecturer in Sociology at City University, London. Paul is interested in the historical development of and inter-relationship between the penal and asylum systems. Paul is involved in service user research (Godin P, Davies J, Heyman B, *et al*. Opening communicative space: a Habermasian understanding of a user-led participatory research project. *J Foren Psych Psychol.* 2007; **18**(4): 452–69). He is also editor and main contributing author to the textbook *Risk and Nursing Practice* (2006) in the Palgrave Sociology and Nursing Practice series.

## PAUL HAYTON

After serving in the Royal Air Force as a pilot, Paul Hayton qualified in health education and health promotion and joined the National Health Service to assist the development of public health, specializing in HIV prevention. In 1997, he was invited to become the first specialist in health promotion in prison health in England and immediately became involved in the management of the WHO Health in Prisons Project. He became Deputy Director of the WHO Collaborating Centre for the Project which is based in the Department of Health, London. The need for further academic work in this field led to his appointment as the Director of the Healthy Prisons program within the Healthy Settings Development Unit, School of Postgraduate Medicine, University of Central Lancashire, UK. One of his most challenging tasks recently has been in developing the national policy for the prison service in England and Wales as regards smoking control.

## JONATHAN HIRST

Between 1993 and 2007, Jonathan Hirst worked as a Youth and Family Counselor with children, youth and families in the areas of child abuse and neglect, mental health, drug and alcohol issues, and youth homelessness. Currently, he is employed by the Victorian Department of Human Services as a lawyer working in the Children's Court. He has a strong interest in the effect on families from the interaction of mental health, drug and alcohol issues, and the legal system.

## KATHLEEN KENDALL

For the last nine years Kathleen Kendall has been teaching sociology in the Medical School at the University of Southampton in the UK. Recently, she has been leading curriculum development and coordinating the first year of the medical degree program. She left Canada in 1993 in order to undertake a PhD at the University of Manchester. Prior to this time, she worked for the Correctional Service of Canada as a Special Advisor on Female Offenders and as a consultant conducting an evaluation of therapeutic service at the Prison for Women in Ontario. Her key research interests are around issues of prisoner mental health.

## DEBBIE KILROY

Debbie Kilroy holds a BSocWk; she has numerous other accomplishments including Psychotherapist, LLB, Order of Australia Medal, and Director of Sisters Inside, a community organization that advocates for the human rights of women in the criminal justice system. Debbie continues to be a strong activist, both nationally and internationally, on issues relating to the abolition of prisons. She is the first former prisoner in Australia to be admitted to practice law.

## LARS MØLLER

Lars Møller is a physician with a specialization in public health medicine. He obtained his doctoral degree in medicine from the University of Copenhagen,

Denmark, and doctorate in Medical Science in 1998. He has done postgraduate work in hospitals and at the Public Health Institute, Copenhagen University. His special interest was in epidemiology and disease prevention and he undertook work for the National Board of Health, the lead department attached to the Ministry of Health on health issues in Denmark. For a number of years, from 1992 until 2001, he was a medical consultant for the International Rehabilitation Council for Torture Victims. He joined the WHO Regional Office for Europe in 2001 and took on the management of its Health in Prisons Project in 2002. Since then, the Project has quickly grown, with 36 European countries participating, and with key advisory publications on the main health issues facing prisons. After some years of development, in 2007 he published *Health in Prisons: a WHO guide to the essentials in prison health*, in English, Russian, Italian and several other languages.

### VIRGINIA OLESEN

As a sociologist in the Department of Social and Behavioral Sciences, School of Nursing, University of California, San Francisco, Virginia Olesen focused on qualitative research and the sociology of health and illness, particularly women's health, and continues to do so. With colleagues she established a Women, Health and Healing emphasis for doctoral students in sociology and nursing. Her publications include: Ruzek S, Olesen V, Clarke A, editors. *Women's Health: complexities and diversities*. Ohio State University Press; 1997, and Clarke A, Olesen V, editors. *Revisioning Women, Health and Healing*. Routledge; 1999.

### JUDY PARKER

Currently Judy Parker works as Professor and Head of the School of Nursing and Midwifery at Victoria University in Melbourne and has previously held positions as Head and/or Professor of Nursing at three other universities. As one of the first PhD prepared nurses working in higher education in Australia, she has spent many years developing the discipline of nursing through teaching programs, research and scholarship. She was honored with an Order of Australia Medal for her services to nursing scholarship and has undertaken substantial work internationally, supporting health care improvements through nursing education and research. She has a strong interest in social justice and enjoys doting on her four grandchildren.

### CINDY PETERNELJ-TAYLOR

As a Professor with the College of Nursing, University of Saskatchewan, Cindy Peternelj-Taylor's career has focused on professional role development for nurses working with vulnerable populations in forensic psychiatric/correctional settings. In this role, she has had opportunities to assist students and nurses with clinical and ethical concerns that emerge from practice. She is a member of the editorial board of the *Journal of Psychiatric and Mental Health Nursing* and an Associate Editor of the *Journal of Forensic Nursing*. She is currently a doctoral candidate with the University of Alberta, where she is completing a dissertation on the experience of nurse engagement with forensic patients in secure environments.

## LISA REYNOLDS

Lisa Reynolds' professional background is in mental health nursing. She has worked extensively in forensic mental health care in the UK, both in secure and community settings. For the past six years she has worked at City University (London) as a lecturer and research fellow. She has been involved with the development of reusable learning objects including an online discussion forum for mental health service users and pre-registration nursing students. She has also supported a forensic mental health service user-led research project in which the service users explored their experiences of forensic mental health care in the UK. Her main research interests are in risk assessment and management, service user involvement and forensic mental health care.

## BETH RICHIE

Beth Richie is a sociologist who has been an activist and an advocate in the movement to end violence against women and against women's incarceration for the past 20 years. The emphasis of her work has been on the ways that race/ethnicity and social position affect women's experience of violence, focusing on the experiences of African-American battered women and sexual assault survivors and women in prison. She has been a trainer and technical assistant to local and national organizations, and frequently lectures to grassroots professionals as well as academic organizations. She is currently an Associate Dean in the College of Liberal Arts and Sciences at the University of Illinois, Chicago. In 2007 she was the recipient of the UIC Woman of the Year Award and recognized with a Faculty Scholars Award. Former Head of the Department of African-American Studies, she is also on the faculty of the Department of Criminal Justice UIC. She is the author of the book *Compelled to Crime: the gender entrapment of battered black women* (Routledge; 1996) and numerous book chapters on women in prison and violence against women. Her new book manuscript is titled *Black Women, Male Violence and the Build Up of a Prison Nation*.

## JANET (JAN) STORCH

Jan Storch began her studies in ethics, law and health care ethics at the University of Alberta, Canada, where she was also a founding member of the Bioethics Centre and taught ethics. Later, as Dean of Nursing at the University of Calgary (Canada) she led the development of a provincial health ethics network (PHEN) for Alberta that continues a strong presence. She studied at the Kennedy Institute of Ethics, following which she became Director of the School of Nursing at the University of Victoria (Canada). At UVIC she found colleagues anxious to engage in nursing ethics research that has continued over the past nine years. She was Ethics Scholar in Residence at the Canadian Nurses Association (CNA), and she has led the past three revisions of the Code of Ethics for Registered Nurses.

## NANCY STOLLER

Nancy Stoller is a research professor at the University of California, Santa Cruz, where she is affiliated with the Community Studies, Sociology and Feminist Studies departments. She has studied health conditions in prisons and jails for over 30 years, with an emphasis on the impact of incarceration on women's health. She is a co-author of the American Public Health Association's *Standards for Health Care in Jails and Prisons* (2003) and currently serves as coordinator of the APHA jail and prisons group.

## DONNA WILLMOTT

Donna Willmott worked as an Advocacy Coordinator at Legal Services for Prisoners with Children in San Francisco for over a decade, working with families of prisoners, community activists and public health experts to counter the devastating effects of incarceration on poor communities and communities of color. She is part of the faculty of the Health Education and Community Health Studies Department of the City College of San Francisco, where she teaches about the health impacts of incarceration.

# CHAPTER 1

# The Ongoing Struggle for Ethical Ideals: Justice and Human Rights

Anne Davis

Ethics is not an ideal system which is all very noble in theory but no good in practice. The reverse of this is closer to the truth: an ethical judgment that is no good in practice must suffer from a theoretical defect as well, for the whole point of ethical judgments is to guide practice.[1]

## INTRODUCTION

Perhaps the first philosopher to use the term "human rights" was Henry David Thoreau in his influential treatise, *Civil Disobedience*. This work influenced many, including Tolstoy, Gandhi, and Martin Luther King, Jr.[2] Thoreau refused to pay his tax because he opposed slavery and the US war against Mexico: as a result the town constable arrested him, and Thoreau spent a night in the city jail for civil disobedience.

Since then many individuals and groups have used this term, human rights, in socio-political debate and action. Today millions of web sites focused on human rights provide insights, including that this ethical and legal ideal is a long-standing, difficult to enforce, humanistic goal not yet fully achieved. However, these sites also tell us that much activity on human rights issues is underway. The sites detail historical facts, recent realities and abuses, and include those run by activist organizations that disclose violations of human rights and advocate for change. Over 23 million web sites focus on rights and prisoners, a vulnerable population with respect to the basic values of liberty, justice, and human rights.

In industrialized countries, some think that human rights violations only occur in other places. However, Amnesty International and similar advocacy groups remind us that this perception is limited and faulty. Believing that human rights violations happen only elsewhere serves as a convenient myth that allows us to dismiss larger socio-ethical issues as not our problem. Additionally, some people think that those deprived of their human rights, whether at home or elsewhere, possibly deserve such treatment given who they are and/or what they have done. This list might include international terrorists and/or citizens who have broken local laws and are now incarcerated. Whatever governments and individuals think about human rights and their violation, these ideals, perceptions and definitions need close and constant examination. The United Nations (UN), numerous national governments, Amnesty International and other groups have made it clear that incarcerated people have human rights and that no person's freedom should be violated without just cause. How "just cause" is determined can be at issue in the law itself and in how the law is enacted.

Human rights transcend formal and informal boundaries but the world is divided by many factors including geography, religion, ethnicity, political systems, gender, and economics. Sometimes a group that is held together by one of these factors comes to define another group, which differs from it, as *The Other*. Sometimes this *Other* becomes defined as sub-human or non-human, making it possible to violate the rights of that group. One does not have to reach far back into history to find this mentality. It continues today. Recent examples include: the Nazis and the Jews; white people and people of color; Protestant and Catholic; Hindu and Muslim; men and women; one tribe and another tribe; people of one country and people of another country.

This chapter has four aims: (1) to explore the philosophical and historical roots of the ethical principle of justice; (2) to define the concept of human rights; (3) to describe briefly the link between health and human rights; and (4) to note selected human rights documents useful in the consideration of justice issues related to the health of incarcerated women.

## MODELS OF JUSTICE

Human rights are grounded in the ethical principle of justice, and several models of justice have been developed that include: (1) formal justice; (2) restorative justice; (3) punitive justice; and (4) social justice. In general, justice has to do with fairness, what is deserved, and to what one is entitled. Formal justice refers to minimal requirement and, according to Aristotle, equals must be treated equally, and unequals must be treated unequally.[3,4] This ethical and legal principle states no criteria for how the notions of equal/unequal are to be determined. Under formal justice, treating similar cases in similar ways and dissimilar cases in dissimilar ways is one of the oldest philosophical truisms. Those who are accused of committing serious crimes are all similar in at least that respect and as a consequence they are treated in similar ways – tried, acquitted or convicted, released or punished (usually) by incarceration in a prison.

Yet there are many differences between these persons that might well be the basis for dissimilar treatment. Traditionally Western penal systems, no doubt under the direct influence of Christianity, were designed primarily for the fallen sinner, the moral agent who had succumbed to temptation but was at least potentially capable of remorse. Eventually this prisoner as penitent became prisoner and debtor, a self-interested person who freely assumed the risk, lost, and now must pay the price. The problem for our society is to match the generic mode of treatment to the criminal. It is very likely that punishment in the strict sense is not a suitable means of dealing with many types of criminals, perhaps only the penitents and the risk-takers. For most of the others, it is pointless or self-defeating.

Restorative justice is concerned with healing victims' wounds, restoring offenders to law-abiding lives, and repairing harm done to interpersonal relationships and the community. This forward-looking, preventive response strives to understand crime in its social context and challenges us to examine root causes of violence and crime.[5-7] This alternative philosophical framework for thinking about crime and criminal justice emphasizes how crime harms relationships in the context of community. Restorative justice gives priority to repairing the harm done to victims, communities, and offenders. In this alternative to punitive justice, both the victim and the community become more actively involved in the justice process. By examining the root causes of crimes committed by women and addressing them, a justice system might be developed that avoids the damage done to all parties and eliminates or reduces the revolving door between community and prison. In this model, only violent career criminals would be imprisoned and those convicted of non-violent crimes would be involved in supervised community projects. This model of criminal justice restores or creates equity and is best accomplished through cooperative processes with all stakeholders involved.[8]

Punitive justice focuses on inflicting punishment and on retribution. Using this model, communities can expel an individual or require that money be paid in damages. This has been the major justice model for much of human history and may be one reason there is a need for an active focus on human rights today. One assumption in this model is that if people are punished for wrongdoings, the public is protected from harm. This is a situation in which individual freedom is greatly limited by the state for the public's safety. Stemming from these notions is the ultimate idea in punitive justice – capital punishment. The evidence, however, does not necessarily support the relationship between the state taking the life of a convicted prisoner and deterring others from committing crimes. For example, in 2004 the Executive Director of the Justice Policy Institute in Washington, DC argued that the drop in crime could not be attributed to tough sentencing laws such as the California "three strikes and you're out" law. Between 1994 and 2002, California's prison system grew by 34724 inmates, while New York's grew by only 315. If tough laws actually protect people, then California's violent crime rate should have dropped relative to New York's. Yet, during this time, New York's violent crime rate dropped 20% more than California's. Schiraldi[9] notes that the problems of crime and the challenges of public safety cannot be solved by draconian laws with catchy names.

Social justice refers to an entire society. It is based on the notion of a just society that gives both individuals and groups fair treatment and a just share of the society's benefits (distributive justice). This model of justice came to prominence at the end of the nineteenth century after 1861 when Mill wrote his famous book on utilitarianism.[10] He believed that societies could be virtuous in the same way that individuals could be. While critics question whether this virtue can be ascribed to today's complex societies,[11] social justice concerns of equity, burdens, and shared benefits, are used by social scientists to critique prisons and their health policies. Some argue that it is a social injustice when incarceration occurs at high rates and with great disparities.[12]

## HUMAN RIGHTS

The complex idea of human rights, based on the fundamental ethical principle of justice, has various definitions. One definition is: human rights are held by all persons equally, universally, and forever. They are inalienable, indivisible and interdependent. Human rights are those basic standards without which people cannot live in dignity. To violate someone's human rights is to treat that person as though he or she were not a human being. To advocate for human rights is to demand that the human dignity of all people be respected.[13]

The most fundamental legal definition of human rights is: the basic rights and freedoms to which all humans are entitled, often held to include the right to life and liberty, freedom of thought and expression, and equality before the law. This definition addresses the role of the state toward the individual and the role of the individual in the state and includes civil, political, economic, social and cultural rights.[14] This idea, equality before the law, has been criticized by some who raise it as a socio-political issue, especially with regard to sentencing individuals in the courts. If justice is blind, the legal system would not and should not discriminate against a person because he or she has certain personal or social attributes such as gender, ethnicity, or social class. However, we know that in some countries poor people are more likely to be incarcerated than those who are economically better off. Langston Hughes, the poet and social critic, wrote:

> That justice is a blind goddess
> Is a thing to which we poor are wise:
> Her bandage hides two festering sores
> That once, perhaps, were eyes.[15]

The question is: can we have the possibility of doing justice in an unjust society?

Rousseau (1712–78) writing about the "Social Contract" contends that all rights are essentially social. Furthermore, law, as the voice of the general will, provides security in human rights. The legal system codifies values and ethics developed over time and provides society with ways of enforcing them. Under the law, liberty is the only human right that is not illusory.[16]

Rights can be thought of as positive rights or liberties and negative rights or liberties. Negative rights, developed mostly from the English/American legal tradition, denote those actions that governments should not take. These are the rights of humans to be left alone and include freedom of religion, speech, and assembly. Positive rights stem from the Rousseauian continental European legal tradition and denote rights that the state has obligation to protect and provide. These rights were codified in the UN Universal Declaration of Human Rights and in numerous national constitutions during the twentieth century.[17]

## SELECTED HISTORY ON JUSTICE AND HUMAN RIGHTS

Any definition of justice and human rights must be understood in the context of its time. Justice and human rights, in some form, are far from new. Both the concept and institutions of human rights have evolved over time and across civilizations to form our present thinking about justice and human rights. That these long-held values are violated in our own time does not render them less important. Indeed, these violations reinforce the need to cherish, advocate, and act to ensure human rights for all.

While not always lived up to or enforced, the ethical and legal concept of justice has a long history in both the East and the West as an ideal fundamental to good society and to which individuals and governments should aspire. Plato (427–347 BCE), a student of and greatly influenced by Socrates, viewed justice as an overarching virtue or character trait of individuals and also basic to the nature of the ideal republic.[18] Aristotle (384–322 BCE) in an analysis of justice described three kinds: (1) distributive; (2) correction; and (3) equity. Justice, a virtue, included lawfulness and fairness and was part of one's motive and one's behavior. Justice had to do with restoring or maintaining a proper balance.[3,4]

The Confucius Analects is a collection of ordered sayings originally embedded in a conversational context within which their meaning could be gradually extracted. Confucius (Kong Fu-zi, 551–479 BCE) saw abuses in China under which people suffered during the feudal system of government and social organization and this led him to develop a moral discipline. Conservative in its adherence to the imperial idea, his moral precepts were intended to teach the Emperor how to use power with justice. His Analects outline five primary virtues: love, justice, reverence, wisdom, and sincerity.[19]

Some religious texts also mention justice although its meaning is not always the same. In the Judeo-Christian Bible both the word "just" and the word "justice" occur. Any detailed description of justice found in the Jewish Torah and the Christian Bible are beyond this chapter due to the complexities surrounding the concept; however, a first principle is: what is hateful to you, do not do to your fellow and the Golden Rule which says, do unto others as you would have them do unto you. In the Christian Bible, the book of Micah 6:8, reads: what does the Lord require of you but to do justice, and to love mercy and to walk humbly with your God.

The Buddhist canonical literature rarely mentions justice. Until the nineteenth century the social order for many Asians presented the same inevitability as the natural order. Mention was made of the proper balanced relations between social groups which show elements of social justice. One reason given for this situation is the importance of the central principle "karma" in Buddhism with the world view of a more fixed universe.[20]

Hinduism says that the excellence of justice consists precisely in the fact that it is compounded of the truth, the good, and the beautiful. The force of a law, a judicial decision, or administrative act depends on the extent of its justice.[21]

In Islam, according to many scholars, one word captures the essence of all of its law and teachings; one word permeates all Islamic values, and that is "justice". In the Islamic holy book, Koran (Qur'an), it is written:

> We sent aforetime our messengers with clear signs and sent down with them the Book and the Balance that all men may stand forth in Justice.[22] (Qur'an Al-Hadeed 57:25)

What is today recognized as the first human rights document, the Cyrus Cylinder, was issued by Cyrus the Great of Persia in the sixth century BCE and established unprecedented principles of human rights. This document abolished slavery and allowed citizens of the empire to practice their religious beliefs freely. These human rights are mentioned in the Biblical books of Chronicles and Ezra.

During the third century BCE in the Mauryan Empire of ancient India, Ashoka the Great established principles of human rights with a policy of non-violence. He also offered free university education to citizens.[20]

In 1215 (CE) King John of England was forced to sign the Magna Carta that embodied some earlier ideas of justice and human rights. Throughout the eighteenth and nineteenth centuries, human rights, as an ethical and legal principle, was discussed in the philosophical literature by Hegel,[23] Kant,[24] Mill,[10] Paine[25] and Wollstonecraft,[26] among others. These discussions played a major role in framing such documents as the United States Declaration of Independence (1776) and the French Declaration of the Rights of Man and Citizens added to the French constitution in 1791. The nineteenth century had slavery, serfdom, inhuman working conditions for adults and children, and starvation wages, among other socio-economic, human rights problems. In our own era, philosophers and social critics continue to write about justice and human rights and voice concerns about vulnerable populations such as the poor, women, children, the mentally ill, and prisoners.[27-30]

## MODERN HUMAN RIGHTS MOVEMENT

The social institution that we know as the modern human rights movement developed from the earlier formation of various groups, usually with specific goals for limited social change. Labor unions fought for the rights of workers; women and some men fought for the rights of women; national liberation movements drove out colonial powers; religious and racial minorities used non-violent methods to gain rights enjoyed by others as a matter of course. In some countries these movements for social change and human rights had the force of a government document that would support the idea of human rights applied to all people regardless of age, gender, social class, political affiliation, religion or ethnicity.

The modern human rights movement stands on the shoulders of many giants past and present, as well as on the shoulders of citizens who may not express their views as often, as publicly or as eloquently but nevertheless constitute a powerful force for social change. Lawyers, journalists, writers and other citizens greatly disturbed by a sentence of 20 years in prison for two Portuguese college students in the UK because they had raised their glasses in a bar to toast "freedom" formed Appeal for Amnesty in 1961. A major London newspaper announced the appeal by referring to six prisoners of conscience from different countries, political, and religious backgrounds jailed for peaceful expressions of their beliefs. A simple plan of action was outlined. The response was more than anyone expected and it grew to become Amnesty International.[31] With this, the modern human rights movement was established internationally. Other such groups focus on human rights and their abuse both at international and national levels. Descriptions of these can be found on numerous web sites. One such group, Human Rights Watch, established in 1978, is comprised of regional watchdog groups to monitor human rights abuses.[32]

These organizations did not create new ethical or legal principles but rather applied established ones to their work. They believe that governments everywhere, regardless of ideology, should create and actively enforce certain basic human rights principles in dealing with their citizens. Recognition of the human rights movement, and especially Amnesty International, increased during the 1970s when Amnesty gained permanent observer status as a non-governmental organization at the UN. Importantly, national governmental bodies around the globe read its reports and its press releases printed in leading newspapers. Amnesty received the Nobel Peace Prize in 1977 for its work on human rights.[31,33]

## HEALTH AND HUMAN RIGHTS

According to experts, health and human rights have three connections: (1) health policies, programs, and practices impact human rights; (2) violations or lack of fulfillment of human rights have negative effects on physical, mental, and social health; and (3) health and human rights act in synergy.[34] The UN Universal Declaration of Human Rights[35] focuses on societal health determinants and provides public health and its practitioners a framework, vocabulary, and guidance for analysis and direct response. Too often health professionals and community leaders such as the clergy and government officials are isolated and removed from the realities of the poor, including those in prisons for minor offenses. These links between human rights and health can serve to lessen, if not eliminate, this isolation. If people concerned with the health of individuals and communities want to move beyond serving the status quo, they must not only understand that the links exist but know how to use them for beneficial purposes. A stronger relationship among the health care sciences (public health, medicine, nursing and social work, etc.), health care ethics, and human rights has developed in recent years in response to the realization that the links between health and human rights are important. Such dramatic reminders as the pandemic of AIDS, SARS, and the possibility of avian flu in humans all point to the need to think and act in both global and local arenas.

We know that poverty does not lead to good health measures but many ethics discussions include only those with access to medical care and medical technology. Health care ethics asks "when is a life worth preserving?" but does not usually include those whose life course is cut short by poverty.[30] Many health professionals have not been at the forefront of changing the factors that link human rights and health since this is not their job. One could argue that many are not equipped to do so, which raises questions about the nature of health care education. Community leaders, as important as they remain, are not always in the vanguard of promoting the link between human rights and health. Do they see the links and, if so, do they do anything about the problems involved?

Human rights and health for women prisoners is the major concern of this book. The penal system offers an ongoing problem in moral justification because it involves the deliberate infliction of harm on people and because it is especially liable to political misuse.[36] Punishment usually is of two kinds: retributive, which claims that punishment is a morally fitting response to criminal offense; and utilitarian, which can be morally justified by appeal to its beneficial effects. Both of these claims in support of moral justification need examination, and especially so for women who have committed minor offenses.

The metaphor used, "war on drugs", denotes potential violence against people, some of whom are viewed in need of help. To justify ethically the incarceration of drug lords and drug pushers is one thing but to imprison drug users raises a myriad of human rights questions in need of ethical analysis.

## HUMAN RIGHTS DOCUMENTS

There are numerous human rights documents with particular pertinence to women prisoners. Some of these documents are overarching while others are specific to this population. All of them can assist in the needed analysis of ethical justifications for incarceration of certain populations such as drug users and the mentally ill.

The values and ethical principles that form the bases of human rights are in documents developed by the UN and various professional associations. Marks[14] compiled a collection of basic international law and policy documents that express the value of human rights for advancing health. Included in this collection are documents from the UN, World Medical Association, and the International Council of Nursing that detail the human rights position on freedom from torture. The section, Right to Health, is central to the concerns in this present book. The documents identify women as a vulnerable population and address human rights issues such as their reproductive rights.

## SUMMARY

This chapter briefly reviewed the ethical and legal principle of justice, the conceptual frame for human rights. Both philosophical and historical support for human rights as a fundamental value was outlined and the interaction between human rights and health was noted. These values of justice and rights for all humans are foundational to the content of this book. Health professionals and others aware of the socio-economic and political human rights issues surrounding the increased imprisonment of women ask: what, if any, gender considerations should influence sentencing? What model of justice would benefit society and individuals? These and other fundamental questions of human rights will be discussed in this book.

## REFERENCES

1 Singer P. About ethics. In: Brosky G, Troyer J, Vance D, editors. *Contemporary Readings in Social and Political Ethics*. Buffalo, NY: Prometheus Books; 1984. p. 9.

2 Thoreau HD. *Civil Disobedience*. Bedford, MA: Applewood Books; 2000.

3 Aristotle. *The Nicomachean Ethics*. New York, NY: Oxford University Press; 1980.

4 Aristotle, Simpson P. *Politics of Aristotle*. Chapel Hill, NC: University of North Carolina Press; 1997.

5 Toews B, Zehr H, editors. *Critical Issues in Restorative Justice*. Monsey, NY: Criminal Justice Press; 2004.

6 Johnstone G. *Restorative Justice: ideas, values, debates*. Devon: Willan Publishing; 2001.

7 Umbreit MS, Coates RB, Kalanj B. *Victim Meets Offender: the impact of restorative justice and mediation*. Monsey, NY: Willow Tree Press; 1994.

8 Zehr H, Mika H. Fundamental concepts of restorative justice. *Contemporary Justice Review.* 1998; 1(1): 47–56.

9 Schiraldi V. To the editor [letter]. *New York Times*. March 19, 2004.

10 Mill JS. *On Liberty and Other Writings*. Cambridge: Cambridge University Press; 1998.

11 Hayek FA. *The Road to Serfdom*. Fiftieth Anniversary Edition. New York, NY: Routledge; 2006.

12 Drucker EM. Incarcerated people. In: Levy BS, Sidel VW, editors. *Social Injustice and Public Health*. Oxford: Oxford University Press; 2006. pp. 161–75.

13 Flowers N. *Human Rights Here and Now: celebrating the Universal Declaration of Human Rights: part 1*. University of Minnesota, Human Rights Resource Center. Available at: http://www1.umn.edu/humanrts/edumat/hreduseries/hereandnow/Part-1/default. htm (accessed January 15, 2009).

14 Marks SP, editor. *Health and Human Rights: basic international documents*. Cambridge, MA: Harvard University Press; 2004.

15 Hughes L. *The Collected Poems of Langston Hughes*. New York, NY: Vintage/Random House; 1995.

16 Rousseau J. *The Social Contract and the Discourses*. New York, NY: Alfred Knopf; 1993.

17 Beauchamp TL, Childress JF. *Principles of Biomedical Ethics*. New York, NY: Oxford University Press; 2001.

18 Cooper JM, Hutchinson DS. *Plato: complete works*. Indianapolis, IN: Hackett Publishing; 1997.

19 Confucius. *Analects: book two*. Indianapolis, IN: Hackett Publishing; 2003.

20 Loy D. *The Great Awakening: a Buddhist social theory*. Somerville, MA: Wisdom Publications; 2003.

21 Hemenway P. *Hindu Gods: the spirit of the divine*. San Francisco, CA: Chronicle Books; 2003.

22 Dawood NJ (translator), editor. *Koran*. New York, NY: Penguin Books; 2003.

23 Hegel GWF. The phenomenology of the spirit. In: Houlgate S, editor. *The Hegel Reader*. Malden, MA: Blackwell; 1998. pp. 45–124.

24 Woods AW, editor. *Basic Writings of Immanuel Kant*. New York, NY: Modern Library; 2001.

25 Paine T. *Common Sense, The Rights of Man, and Other Essential Writings.* New York, NY: Penguin Books; 2003.

26 Wollstonecraft M. *A Vindication of the Rights of Women (1792).* New York, NY: Dover; 1996.

27 Rawls J. *A Theory of Justice.* Cambridge, MA: Harvard University Press; 1971.

28 Sen A. *Development as Freedom.* New York, NY: Random House; 1999.

29 Nussbaum M. *Sex and Social Justice.* New York, NY: Oxford University Press; 1999.

30 Farmer P. *Pathologies of Power: health, human rights, and the new war on the poor.* Berkeley, CA: University of California Press; 2003.

31 Power J. *Like Water on Stone: the story of Amnesty International.* Boston, MA: Northeastern University Press; 2001.

32 Human Rights Watch. *About Us.* Available at: www.hrw.org/about/whoweare.html. (accessed February 23, 2009).

33 Clark AM. *Diplomacy of Conscience: Amnesty International and changing human rights norms.* Princeton, NJ: University Press; 2001.

34 Mann JM, Gruskin S, Grodin MA, *et al.*, editors. *Health and Human Rights: a reader.* New York, NY: Routledge; 1999.

35 United Nations. *The Universal Declaration of Human Rights.* 2008. Available at: www.un.org/events/humanrights/udhr60/index.shtml (accessed January 15, 2009).

36 Brodsky G, Troyer J, Vance D. *Contemporary Readings in Social and Political Ethics.* Buffalo, NY: Prometheus Books; 1984.

# CHAPTER 2

# Social Capital: A Lens for Examining Health of Incarcerated and Formerly Incarcerated Women

Virginia Olesen

The worrisome and enduring health problems among women prisoners, though thoughtfully examined in numerous excellent reports,[1-5] demand fresh perspectives if policy makers and practitioners are to address them successfully. To that end this chapter examines social capital, widely used in the social sciences and public health, as a perspective to facilitate rethinking these grievous problems to realize change. It attempts to make abstract social science thinking relevant to a pressing human problem, recognizing that the complexity of human affairs often can and does exceed what science conceptualizes. Complexity acknowledged, it is nevertheless worthwhile to harness such concepts to the task of generating different perspectives and critical outlooks on obdurate problems. This approach analyzes the situation as it is, recognizing that many aspects of women prisoners' health, such as the problem of overcrowding due to substantial increases in numbers of imprisoned women,[6-10] are issues that beg for judicial and prison reform, topics for another analysis.

I will first discuss social capital, its history, dimensions, strengths and weaknesses, to clarify and deconstruct the concept. This sets up a discussion on social capital and health and, more specifically, social capital and health of women during and after incarceration. Finally, I note some implications of social capital for thinking about and acting on these issues.

## SOCIAL CAPITAL, THE CONCEPT

Social capital can be understood as "the ability of actors to secure benefits by virtue of membership in social networks or other social structures."[11(p.6)] (For literate and informative reviews, *see* 11–14.) Social capital has two critical elements: the social relationships that allow individuals access to resources possessed by their associates; and the amount and quality of those resources.[11(pp.3,4)] Simply being a member of a network does not assure an individual access to resources, if the network members have no or few resources. Though some recent formulations have extended the idea of social capital to communities,[14(p.117)] in the interests of closely examining health of women during and after incarceration, this chapter primarily focuses on: (a) individual access and relationship to networks; and (b) the resources and associates in those networks. Because social capital derives from the interactions in networks,[15] this chapter's focus takes note of feminist criticisms that conceptualizations of social capital need to be embedded in social relations shaped by gender, class, race, age, and sexual orientation,[16] rather than ignoring women or simply adding them in.[13,17,18]

## NETWORKS

To discuss how social interaction within networks accesses social capital, it is useful to characterize the ties in those networks. This brief outline relies on the useful discussion in Ferlander.[14]

Networks can be characterized by the direction of the ties in the network (vertical or horizontal), their levels of formality (formal or informal), and their strength (weak or strong). For example, *formal and horizontal ties* include voluntary associations; *informal and horizontal ties* include family, friends, neighbors, and colleagues; *formal and vertical ties* include church and work hierarchies; *informal and vertical ties* include criminal networks, clan relations, and street gangs.

Networks can also be depicted by level of strength, diversity, direction, and their function (bonding, bridging, linking). For example: *bonding with strong horizontal ties* includes close friends and family with similar social characteristics; *bonding with weak horizontal ties* includes members with similar interests or characteristics in voluntary associations; *bridging with strong horizontal ties* includes close friends and family with different social characteristics; *bridging with weak horizontal ties* includes acquaintances and members with different social characteristics in voluntary associations; *linking with strong vertical ties* includes close work colleagues with different hierarchical positions; *linking with weak vertical ties* includes distant colleagues with different hierarchical positions, such as ties between citizens and civil servants. Different networks yield different access to or denial of social capital. Strong and bonding networks provide instrumental and emotional support, but may also exclude others.[19] Weak and bridging ties can provide information not always available in the networks of intimates with strong bonding.

Not surprisingly, social inequality characterizes networks and the access they provide to social capital. Because individuals tend to associate with others having similar characteristics, those in resource-rich networks have greater variety of resources, including information, in contrast to those in resource-poor networks.[20] In other words, to use the old phrase, "them's as has, gits." Issues of gender and race further complicate this: ". . . females are affiliated with disadvantaged networks, more female ties, [and] ties in lower hierarchical positions."[20(p.788)] Research also notes a similar lack of access to social capital among ethnic and racial minorities embedded in resource-poor networks.[20] In sum, social capital is a resource, accessed through networks. How then is it related to health issues?

## SOCIAL CAPITAL AND HEALTH

Despite misgivings about the conceptualization of social capital,[18,21-4] numerous analyses (more than 800 from a Web of Science search) have utilized social capital in its various iterations to examine health issues. A few are summarized here: Campbell examined social capital to understand relations between health and deprivation;[25] Kawachi and Berkman demonstrated possible pathways between social capital and health;[15] Cattell and Herring learned that social capital has benefits for health, but must be considered in the political, economic context of people's lives and the resilience of their communities;[26] Liukkonen, *et al.* found partial support for the idea that work-related social capital (co-worker support) is a health resource;[27] Kritsotakis and Gamarnikow argued that trust is related to social capital in relation to health;[23] and Almedon's work showed that meaningful examination of social capital scrutinizes individual access to, rather than possession of, social capital.[28]

Ferlander reviewed the connections between types of networks and health.[14] She noted that much health care research demonstrates the positive relationship between health and strong, horizontal, informal social networks, but also points to negative relationships of strong, bonding networks, such as stress for overburdened members of deprived communities who try to meet difficult obligations. She underscored the importance of mutuality in various networks, an under-examined topic in health and social capital. Where unhealthy practices or behaviors occur, strong bonding networks may result in risky behaviors, an indication of "the human tendency to follow one's peers."[14(p.122)] Representing contact with non-intimate others, weak bridging and linking networks improve chances for contacts with potentially helpful others and new information not available in tight, bonded networks.

## INCARCERATED AND FORMERLY INCARCERATED WOMEN, HEALTH AND SOCIAL CAPITAL

With few exceptions[4,29] the concept of social capital has not been widely used to analyze women during and after incarceration, perhaps because of the concept's continually evolving status and its complexity (bridging networks; ties; structural, interactional and emotional issues). Lacking such analyses, it is still possible to scrutinize research reports, policy documents, and personal accounts about health of women prisoners using social capital as a lens to discover and recover elements relevant to social capital in these sources. In other words one can do an exploratory analysis using social capital as a sensitizing code. I will use this strategy, found in qualitative research,[30] to examine a few promising reports on women prisoners and their health, since the literature is more extensive than this chapter can cover. This is not a substitute for well-funded, well-articulated qualitative and quantitative research, and humane, practical policies based on such inquiries. It is an intermediate tactic to explore application of an abstract social science concept to obdurate, real-world problems.

### Social Capital and Health of Imprisoned Women

Thoughtful inquiries about women prisoners' health and services for them have generally yielded dismal pictures of neglect and, in some instances, abuse.[3,31–33] The substantial health problems with which many women enter prison, including mental illness, substance abuse, prior poor health, and chronic illnesses,[4,6] are often exacerbated by the stresses of imprisonment, such as loss of contact with children, abuse and neglect in prison.[3] Even though some claim their health improved while they were incarcerated,[34] many depart prison less "healthy" than they were upon entry.[35,36] Major factors contribute to their poor health, including the inadequacy of health care services and lack of access to care.[2,32]

Adequate health care services for imprisoned women are an important resource, and policies that improve the quality of and access to care are urgently needed. The networks through which women prisoners access resources are relevant to issues of health and health care. First-hand accounts from women prisoners vividly detail the importance of close relationships for emotional and social support and, by implication, accessing resources: "I had a few really good friends I met in prison and the funny thing is these girls would do anything for you."[3(p.536)] At the same time some prisoners' accounts reveal that there are networks and relationships wherein access to resources comes at a very high price of personal physical and mental abuse.[3] Other prisoners' comments suggest that interpersonal relationships may not always be trustworthy.[37]

Imprisoned women remain part of networks on the outside, but their confinement isolates them, and family structures often weaken during incarceration.[38] Ties to family and friends are reduced,[39] particularly when visits are infrequent. One study found that although more than half the women studied received phone calls or mail from families, more than half of imprisoned mothers had none or only one or two visits while incarcerated.[40] Hence their participation in and contribution to networks where mutuality is critical in accessing social capital are diminished. Nevertheless, many imprisoned women do try to access networks as they attempt to provide for care of children, and to reconcile with partners and/or other family members. In sum, the concept of social capital offers a way to look at imprisoned women's networks and health, even where services are less than adequate.

### Social Capital and Health of Women Leaving Prison

Women released from prison face formidable challenges in finding stable, safe housing, treatment for continuing health problems, employment, and reunion with children and families.[5,34] These valuable health-related resources are, of course, not available to all. Accessing them through networks may be highly problematic, as networks are unevenly distributed across social groups.[29] Variations exist among formerly incarcerated women with regard to size of networks and available support: better educated women have larger networks, hence more chances for emotional, social, instrumental, and general support in contrast to low income or poorly educated women.[29] Younger women are members of networks with lower levels of support.[29] Thus, many women departing prison return to networks that are poor in social capital,[29] instances of what this chapter earlier pointed to as strong, bonding networks – horizontal ties to families and friends with less diversity in contacts, and offering little in the way of information or skills to achieve acquisition of resources. Even with strong, bonding networks where limited social capital may exist, access to resources may be difficult because others in the network may shun or marginalize a former prisoner because of the stigmatized status of "ex-con."[34(p.383)]

## DISCUSSION

The role of networks in accessing resources can deepen our analysis of the health of women prisoners. However, emphasizing networks in no way avoids the necessity to explore and act on the urgent issues of providing adequate care for imprisoned women.[2,32,41,42] Nor does it sidestep the critical need for programs that facilitate resources for released women.[4,34,43,44] Above all it does not overlook that situations to which many imprisoned women return are highly deprived, resource-poor contexts with impoverished networks, particularly for poorly educated and young women. Alleviating poverty and its invidious sequelae are critical agendas beyond the scope of this chapter.

Emphasizing networks acknowledges the importance of crucial resources found in prison reform and release programs, and raises the question of how such are accessed through women's networks while in prison and upon community reentry. Thinking back to the outline of types of networks noted earlier, even in prison women are members of several types of networks that yield differential access to resources. It should not be assumed that all women are members of only one type of network. Given the constraints of prison life and what is known about "prison families"[45] it is likely that many women are in bonding networks with strong, horizontal ties involving family and friends. Yet even in prison there may be the possibility of weak, horizontal or vertical ties that yield information and resources. Exploration of those networks and their relationship to health would be very useful as a way to understand how to enhance women's access to health-related resources. Given the difficult complexities of prison life for women, however, this would require careful, ethical research, involving prisoners themselves as participants in the research process, not merely as "subjects." Although not easy, this type of inquiry could prove valuable in expanding understanding of how networks, even in a difficult situation, enhance or deter women's access to health care resources.

Consideration of how different types of networks may be in play at the same time for their members is another important contribution to developing a more precise understanding of the relationships between social capital and health. The finding that paroled women who participate in community programs have more social capital is instructive.[29] Perhaps this is because community programs afford more diverse contexts and contacts or, to return to the earlier conceptualization of networks, they function as bridge networks with weak social ties, which can provide more information, and other resources. If this is the case then it would be important to put in place programs that facilitate building bridge networks, particularly for younger and more poorly educated former prisoners who have impoverished networks.[29] It is naïve to think that programs alone can build networks, but it is not unrealistic to support programs that enhance network building, particularly those that foster contact with different ties and characteristics, including weak ties that open greater access to resources. These could also enhance mutuality with the recognition that women released to the community, though facing enormous and difficult challenges to stabilize themselves, their families, and their lives, can be and are active agents, not passive bystanders, in the creation and acquisition of social capital, limited though it might be.

## SUMMARY

Through an examination of the concept of social capital and the situation of incarcerated and formerly incarcerated women, this chapter has attempted to show how women's health can be productively explored by focusing on the importance of networks in realizing social capital.[46] This focus takes an abstract concept into pragmatic realms where fresh approaches are requisite if we are to move to more humane and more productive situations for women prisoners.

## REFERENCES

1 Shaw N. Female prisoners view their health. *J Prison Health: Medicine, Law, Corrections, Ethics.* 1981; **1**(1): 30–43.

2 Ammar NH, Erez E. Health care delivery systems in women's prisons: the case of Ohio. *Federal Probation.* 2000; **64**(1): 19–26.

3 Pogrebin M, Dodge M. Women's accounts of their prison experiences: a retrospective view of their subjective realities. *J Crim Justice.* 2001; **29**: 531–41.

4 Willmott D, van Olphen J. Challenging the health impacts of incarceration: the role for community health workers. *Californian J Health Promot.* 2005; **3**(2): 38–48.

5 Schram P, Koons-Witt B, Williams F, *et al.* Supervision strategies and approaches for female parolees: examining the link between unmet needs and parolee outcome. *Crime Delinq.* 2006; **52**(3): 450–71.

6 Mullings J. Victimization, substance abuse and high risk behavior as predictors of health among women at admission to prison. *Dissertation Abstracts International Section A: Humanities and Social Sciences.* 1998; **58**(9-A): 3730.

7 Kruttschnitt C, Gartner R. Women's imprisonment. *Crime and Justice.* 2003; **30**: 1–81.

8 Langston S. Commentary: the reality of women of color in the prison system. *Journal of Ethnicity in Criminal Justice.* 2003; **1**(2): 85–93.

9 Sokoloff N. Women prisoners at the dawn of the 21st century. *Women Crim Justice.* 2005; **16**(1–2): 127–37.

10 Sudbury J, editor. *Global Lockdown: race, gender, and the prison-industrial complex.* New York, NY: Routledge; 2005.

11 Portes A. Social capital, its origins and applications in modern sociology. *Annu Rev Sociol.* 1998; **24**: 1–24.

12 Schuller T, Baron S, Field J. Social capital, a review and critique. In: Baron S, Field J, Schuller T, editors. *Social Capital: critical perspectives.* Oxford: Oxford University Press; 2000. pp. 1–38.

13 Field J, Schuller T, Baron S. Social capital and human capital revisited. In: Baron S, Field J, Schuller T, editors. *Social Capital: critical perspectives.* Oxford: Oxford University Press; 2000. pp. 243–63.

14 Ferlander S. The importance of different forms of social capital for health. *Acta Sociol.* 2007; **50**(2): 115–28.

15 Kawachi I, Berkman L. Social cohesion, social capital and health. In: Berkman L, Kawachi I, editors. *Social Epidemiology.* Oxford: Oxford University Press; 2000. pp. 174–90.

16 Franklin J, Thomson R. (Re)claiming the social: a conversation between feminist, late modern, and social capital theories. *Feminist Theory.* 2005; **6**(2): 161–72.

17 Kovalainen A. Rethinking the revival of social capital and trust in social theory: possibilities for feminist analysis. In: Marshall B, Witz A, editors. *Engendering the Social:*

*feminist encounters with social theory*. Maidenhead, England: Open University Press; 2004. pp. 155–70.

18 Bezanson K. Gender and the limits of social capital. *Can Rev Sociol Anthropol.* 2006; **43**(4): 427–44.

19 Portes A, Landolt P. The downside of social capital. *Am Prospect.* 1996; **26**: 18–23.

20 Lin N. Inequality in social capital. *Contemporary Sociology.* 2000; **29**(6): 785–95.

21 Adkins L. Social capital: the anatomy of a troubled concept. *Feminist Theory.* 2005; **6**(2): 195–211.

22 Carlson ED, Chamberlain RM. Social capital, health and health disparities. *J Nurs Scholarsh.* 2003; **35**(4): 325–31.

23 Kritsotakis G, Gamarnikow E. What is social capital and how does it relate to health? *Int J Nurs Stud.* 2004; **41**(1): 43–50.

24 Misztal B. The new importance of the relationship between formality and informality. *Feminist Theory.* 2005; **6**(2): 172–94.

25 Campbell C. Social capital and health: contextualizing health promotion within local community efforts. In: Baron S, Field J, Schuller T, editors. *Social Capital: critical perspectives.* Oxford: Oxford University Press; 2000. pp. 182–96.

26 Cattell V, Herring R. Social capital and well-being: generations in an East London neighbourhood. *Journal of Mental Health Promotion.* 2002; **1**(3): 8–19.

27 Liukkonen V, Virtanen P, Kivimaki M, *et al.* Social capital in working life and the health of employees. *Soc Sci Med.* 2004; **59**(12): 2447–58.

28 Almedon AM. Social capital and mental health: an interdisciplinary review of primary evidence. *Soc Sci Med.* 2005; **61**(5): 943–64.

29 Reisig M, Holtfreter K, Morash M. Social capital among women offenders: examining the distribution of social networks and resources. *J Contemp Crim Justice.* 2002; **18**(2): 167–87.

30 Strauss AL. *Qualitative Analysis for Social Scientists.* Cambridge: Cambridge University Press; 1987.

31 Acoca L. Defusing the time bomb: understanding and meeting the growing health care needs of incarcerated women in America. *Crime Delinq.* 1998; **44**(1): 49–69.

32 Stoller N. *Improving Access to Health Care for California's Women Prisoners.* Berkeley, CA: California Policy Research Center, University of California; 2001. Available at: http://cpac.berkeley.edu/documents/stollerpaper.pdf (accessed May 24, 2009).

33 Stoller N. Space, place and movement as aspects of health care in three women's prisons. *Soc Sci Med.* 2003; **56**(11): 2263–75.

34 Richie B. Challenges incarcerated women face as they return to their communities: findings from life history interviews. *Crime Delinq.* 2001; **47**(3): 368–89.

35 Freudenberg N. Adverse effects of US jail and prison policies on the health and well-being of women of color. *Am J Public Health.* 2002; **92**(12): 1895–9.

36 Freudenberg N, Daniels J, Crum M, *et al.* Coming home from jail: the social and health consequences of community reentry for women, male adolescents, and their families and communities. *Am J Public Health.* 2005; **95**(10): 1725–36.

37 Greer K. The changing nature of interpersonal relationships in a women's prison. *Prison J.* 2000; **80**(4): 442–68.

38 Sharp S, Marcus-Mendoza S. It's a family affair: incarcerated women and their families. *Women Crim Justice.* 2001; **12**(4): 21–49.

39 Visher C, Travis J. Transitions from prison to community: understanding individual pathways. *Annu Rev Sociol.* 2003; **29**: 89–113.

40 Arditti JA, Few AL. Mothers' reentry into family life after incarceration. *Criminal Justice Policy Review.* 2006; **17**(1): 103–23.

41 Sobel S. Difficulties experienced by women in prison. *Psychol Women Q.* 1982; **7**(2): 107–18.

42 Kane M, DiBartolo M. Complex physical and mental health needs of rural incarcerated women. *Issues Ment Health Nurs.* 2002; **23**(3): 209–29.

43 Richie BE, Freudenberg N, Page J. Reintegrating women leaving jail into urban communities: a description of a model program. *J Urban Health.* 2001; **78**(2): 290–303.

44 Parsons ML, Warner-Robbins C. Factors that support women's successful transition to the community following jail/prison. *Health Care Women Int.* 2002; **23**: 6–18.

45 Huggins D, Capeheart L, Newman E. Deviants or scapegoats: an examination of pseudofamily groups and dyads in two Texas prisons. *Prison J.* 2006; **86**(1): 114–39.

46 Olesen V, Clarke A. Resisting closure, embracing uncertainties, creating agendas. In: Clarke A, Olesen V, editors. *Revisioning Women, Health and Healing: feminist, cultural and technoscience perspectives.* New York, NY: Routledge; 1999. pp. 355–8.

# CHAPTER 3

# Challenges Incarcerated Women Face as They Return to Their Communities: Findings From Life History Interviews[*]

Beth Richie

Intellectual and public policy discussions regarding prisoner reentry, probation or parole services, and the impact of incarceration on community life more generally, have failed to incorporate the specific challenges that incarcerated women face as they return to their communities. Reflecting the broader relative invisibility of women in the field of criminology and the criminal justice literature, the lack of knowledge about (and perhaps interest in) gender as an important variable in reentry has significantly limited intervention initiatives. This chapter is an attempt to begin to fill this gap by analyzing data about incarcerated women's reentry experiences collected in a series of qualitative studies. A demographic profile of women in jails and prisons in the US will be followed by a discussion of findings from interviews conducted with incarcerated and formerly incarcerated women about the challenges they face upon release from correctional facilities. This discussion will incorporate the analysis of their accounts, a review of the relevant literature, and an evaluation of the gender-related, culturally specific issues that arise from considerations of the broader social and institutional context. The chapter will conclude with research and policy implications.

## PROFILE OF WOMEN IN JAILS AND PRISONS

Although women constitute a small fraction of the total population involved in the criminal justice system in the US, the number of arrests and incarcerations

---

[*]Reprinted with permission. *Crime Delinq.* 2001; 47(3): 368–89.

of women is growing at rates significantly higher than for men. In 1998, 3.2 million women were arrested, accounting for 22% of all the arrestees that year. Women constituted 16% of all people detained in correctional facilities; more than 75 000 are in state prisons, close to 10 000 are in federal facilities, and 64 000 are in US jails. Overall, an estimated 950 000 women are under the care, custody, and control of correctional agencies (including probation and parole) on any given day in the US.[1] Currently, 1.3 million children younger than 18 have mothers under correctional supervision.[2]

Increasingly, women who are incarcerated in the US are there for non-violent, drug-related offenses that account for the largest source of the total growth among female inmates (38% nationally). In some states, the growth has been very dramatic. In New York state, for example, the number of women arrested for drug offenses increased by 98% between 1986 and 1995, convictions by 256%, and prison sentences by 478%.[3] The combined effects of harsh drug laws, changing patterns of drug use, and mandatory sentencing policies have led to a significant boom in women's incarceration rates. Overall, women in jail in 1998 were there for property crimes (31.7%), drug offenses (27.4%), public order crimes (24.7%), violent offenses (14.9%), and other offenses (1.2%).[1]

The racial/ethnic profile of women in jails and prisons represents one of the most vivid examples of racial disparity in American society. By far the majority of women who are incarcerated in the US are women of color. Nearly two-thirds of those confined in jails and state and federal prisons are black, Hispanic, or of other (non-white) ethnic groups.

> The most recent BJS estimate of the lifetime chance of being sent to Federal or State prison at least once indicates that overall about 11 women out of 1,000 will be incarcerated at some time in their lives. The estimates further show that about 5 out of 1,000 white women, 36 out of 1,000 black women, and 15 out of 1,000 Hispanic women will be subjected to imprisonment during their lifetime.[1(p.11)]

Incarcerated women are also young and poor. The median age of the population of women incarcerated in the US is 35. Typically, when they were arrested they were living in low-income communities where they experience many of the difficulties associated with contemporary urban poverty. Less than 40% of women in state prisons report they had been employed full-time prior to arrest, and about 35% had incomes less than $600 per month. Only 39% had a high school diploma or general equivalency diploma (GED). Typically, they come from communities where rates of homelessness have increased substantially, reaching 40% in some studies of women detained in US jails.[4,5]

Data concerning the health and mental health status of incarcerated women reveal that at least 60% of women in state prisons reported a history of physical or sexual abuse.[1] Other studies of abuse history reveal a much higher rate and indicate that the nature of the abuse in this population is particularly severe.[6,7] Other serious health indicators include high rates of HIV positive status (3.5% overall and as high as 25% in some large urban jail populations) and high rates of other sexually transmitted diseases, both of which leave women in compromised health and constant pain.[1,8–10]

The specific health consequences of substance abuse are considerable for the population of women who are most likely to be arrested in the US. Fifty percent of all incarcerated women report that they were using drugs or alcohol at the time of their arrest,[1] and most associate chronic problems with their long-term drug or alcohol addiction. Whereas some studies show that women are initially lured into the illegal drug economy in an attempt to earn money,[11] many end up with serious and debilitating substance abuse problems.[12]

A review of the literature suggests that most of the women who are released from jail or prison are likely to return to the same disenfranchised neighborhoods and difficult conditions without having received any services to address their underlying problems.[13–15] In most of their communities, there are few services and very limited resources available to assist women in the process of reentry.[16] Typically, they face considerable hardships, difficult circumstances, and insufficient opportunities for stabilization. Despite the fact that some women do quite well putting their lives back together when they are released from prison, many return to very precarious situations that may compel them to engage in further illegal activities. In most follow-up studies, prior arrest history was the most important predictor of post-prison recidivism. Sixty-five percent of women confined in state prisons had a history of prior conviction; half had three or more prior convictions.[1]

This statistical picture points clearly to the critical role that neighborhood development and reintegration services could play in decreasing women's recidivism and increasing their chances for successful reentry into their communities. However, there is very little qualitative research that explores the specific, nuanced conditions or the particular circumstances that influence the disturbingly high rate of recidivism for women. As the following discussion will show, an analysis of women's stories offers critical insight into the patterns of incarceration and release, for behind the high rates of arrest and rearrest, there are profoundly troubling and illustrative accounts of institutional and individual failures that threaten successful reintegration for women released from jail or prison in the US.

## NEEDS OF WOMEN RETURNING TO THEIR COMMUNITIES FROM JAIL OR PRISON

The data presented in this chapter are drawn from a series of qualitative research projects designed to explore the causes and consequences of arrest and incarceration for women of color who live in low-income communities. I conducted 42 in-depth interviews using an open-ended instrument and analyzed the data using the grounded-theory method. The findings were coded by theme and then considered in relationship to the relevant literature. The respondents in this sample represent the demographic profile described in the previous section; all have been arrested and released at least three times to disenfranchised neighborhoods where they faced significant challenges to successful reentry. Although the sample size was small and not statistically or randomly selected, the women interviewed represent the demographics and conditions experienced by a population of incarcerated women in the US, and the themes they describe are consistent with past findings.

The thematic patterns described in this chapter focus on how neighborhood conditions, community resources, and public policies affect women's ability to successfully reintegrate into their community upon release from jail or prison. In the aggregate, the findings paint a profoundly complex and disturbing picture. They show how the identical, overwhelming problems women faced prior to entering the system meet them when they leave the jail or prison. An analysis of their accounts revealed seven thematic challenges and barriers to successful reentry to their communities.

### Treatment for Substance Abuse Problems

As indicated previously, most of the women incarcerated in the US are there for drug-related crimes, and most of them have histories of serious long-term substance abuse problems.[17] Whereas many correctional institutions in the US offer some substance abuse intervention programs for inmates, only a small percentage of women inmates who need them have access to chemical dependency treatment programs. Of those women who were able to complete drug treatment while they were incarcerated, many I interviewed reported that short-term, prison-based intervention (in a setting where drugs are not as readily available) does not adequately prepare them to abstain from substance abuse or manage their addiction once they are released into the community.[18] Three key factors emerged from interviews as particularly problematic: lack of access to drug treatment programs; inconclusive evaluations of program effectiveness; and "unnatural" treatment settings.

> Inside, there were some treatment groups, but they only met every once in awhile. I'd try to get there, but sometimes the officers forgot to call me out of

my housing area. Or, I'd get there and the group would be canceled for some reason. Other times, we'd just be there talking, but not getting very deep. It was good to get a distraction, but I wouldn't say I worked on my issues. I'm an addict and have been for eight years. I really need help, but didn't get it in jail. So when I came out, I went right back [to drug abuse]. Nothing changed. And even though I stopped using while I was locked up, that was just because I couldn't use there. I wish I could have used my time [in jail] better 'cause there certainly isn't any programs in the streets. Now I'm back where I started. Running the streets, chasing that drug until I get locked up again. (32-year-old woman serving six years in state prison)

Advocates and service providers agree that substance abuse treatment is one of the most significant needs for women returning to their communities from jails and prisons.

Further exploration of this issue indicates that the programmatic nature of community-based substance abuse treatment is critical to women's successful reintegration. Women described how essential attention to gender-specific needs (such as child care and protection from sexual harassment) is to their ability to enter and complete substance abuse treatment. Given the evidence that relapse is one of the most salient factors in women's recidivism, attention to gender-specific factors is very important in helping women maintain their sobriety over time.[4,19]

I really tried this time to go to treatment. But I couldn't stand how they treated me. Mostly it was the men in the group who always want to get some [have sex]. They offer nicely at first, then they teased me, they just stared at me whenever I talked. It was impossible to ignore their stares. Do you know one even offered to get high with me if I'd give him some [sex]? So I stopped going altogether. (27-year-old woman detained in urban jail)

## Health Care

Medical problems and health care needs were among the most common challenges described during the interviews. Like most women who have been arrested, the sample I interviewed entered correctional facilities with serious medical problems. Yet, despite the mandated presence of health care services in most jails and prisons, many women are released with their health needs unmet. In particular, the women I interviewed described the need for treatment related to complications of HIV, asthma, diabetes, hypertension, and reproductive health problems. Such treatment is paramount for their successful return to the community, because their medical needs are often serious and urgent, presenting serious barriers to reintegration.

> I've been in the hospital four times since last year with one thing or another. I have AIDS, TB and need to have an operation for tumors in my belly because I bleed all the time. Each time, I just keep getting worse and worse because I can't keep up with all of the medicine I am supposed to be taking. Last time, I almost died. It is really messing with me . . . both my mind and my body. If I could just get some of this under control, then I could work on finding a place to live and finding a job. But I am just so sick all the time now. (33-year-old woman detained in an urban jail)

In addition to urgent needs for care, the long-term consequences of drug and alcohol abuse, chronic poor nutrition, and untreated minor health problems (such as dental problems) significantly complicated the women's health and well-being once they were released from correctional facilities. Some data point to a minor overall improvement in the health status of women while they are in jail or prison when compared to their health status upon entering, and most of the women I interviewed did, in fact, report a temporary improvement in their health status while incarcerated. However, the long-term impact of having access to prison or jail health clinics is minimal.[20]

> I was sick as a dog when I came in. I have asthma and problems with my blood pressure since I was a child. My skin was peeling badly, and my sugar [diabetes] was out of control. I was really in bad shape; hungry, tired, cold and sick. After a few days, I started to feel better, I think because I got some medicine for my infections. But as soon as I got out, I got sick again. I don't know what medicine they were giving me, so I can't get a refill. I don't have a doctor, I don't have any money, and I don't know what to do. (21-year-old woman living in a homeless shelter)

That is, whereas some women have access to emergency medical care while they are incarcerated, they typically do not have ongoing attention to their long-term health needs. Without help to manage chronic disease, health problems inevitably follow incarcerated women back to the community once they are released from jail or prison.

## Mental Health Issues

Increasingly, researchers and mental health practitioners are focusing on the relationship between mental health problems and women's involvement in illegal activity. Although the rates of diagnosed mental health conditions may be increasing in the population of women who are incarcerated in this country, advocates and practitioners who work with incarcerated women argue that the actual dimension of the problem is far more serious than even the alarming new statistics would indicate.[21,22] I was impressed by the extent to which the women I interviewed suffered from mental health problems. The majority of them described how even acute major psychological problems were not diagnosed, let alone cases of depression, behavioral disorders, or learning and developmental disabilities. Without any treatment in prison, the women return to their communities with serious and persistent diagnostic and treatment needs for mental health problems. When these needs continue to be unmet, they pose serious barriers to successful reintegration into their communities. More than half of the women interviewed described chronic emotional problems for which they had never received treatment.

> I have had mood problems all of my life. I hear voices at times, and I black out without knowing where I have been. Sometimes I feel so badly, I want to die. Yes, I've tried to kill myself and I am not ashamed to show you these cuts on my arms. It's the voices that tell me to do it. I know it would make my family feel really sad, but it is the only way I can think to solve my problems. (26-year-old woman detained in a secured drug treatment facility)
>
> I have the kind of emotional problems where I just lose my temper and start banging my head against the wall. Sometimes it gets so bad that I stay in bed for a week, just to not hurt myself or someone else. I'm good for awhile, then I fall back into that real deep sadness. (27-year-old woman serving three years in state prison)
>
> I have gone crazy three times before where I have to take pills to get my sanity back. I don't know what the pills are, but when I can get them, they help me not to zone out and run away from reality. That's why I live mostly on the streets; because I zone out and can't find my way back home. (39-year-old woman detained in urban jail)

In the interviews, the women reported periods of disorientation, depression, forgetfulness, and otherwise compromised functioning like those described above. Although I did not know the precise nature of the emotional problems (most could not specify a diagnosis), to me the women's accounts represented troubling evidence of chronic emotional difficulties that seriously limited their ability to function in their community before and especially after their incarceration.

### Violence Prevention and Post-Traumatic Stress Disorder (PTSD)

Women interviewed for this research described how horrific early childhood abuse and extensive adult intimate violence had a profound impact on their lives, including their illegal activity. Although related to the health and mental health needs the women described, evidence of trauma and PTSD was so significant that I coded and analyzed it as a distinct theme. This pattern has been established by other research,[1,6,7] and with other (non-prison) populations it has shown that this type of trauma has long-term consequences that become worse when left untreated.[23] Given the lack of attention to PTSD and violence issues in most correctional settings, it should be expected that women returning from jails and prisons will continue to have unresolved issues related to trauma and abuse.

> I was seriously tripping [having a flashback] when I got arrested. The officer put his hands on me, and I went right back to the last time I was raped. And I fought like hell. I wasn't ever going to let a man touch me like that again. So I kicked him and tried to grab his gun and if I'd gotten it, I would have shot him. I know I would have. Ever since I've been here, I can't trust anyone. If someone moves towards me too fast, I'll just go off. And then I have nightmares all night long. I spend most of my time alone or in the bing [solitary confinement] because I just can't get along with people any more. (21-year-old woman detained in urban jail)

In addition to the more psychologically oriented set of issues, the women I interviewed described very basic needs for safety and protection from further abuse upon release. Their accounts suggest that even though women in abusive relationships are incarcerated (and theoretically protected from physically violent partners on the outside) they continue to be controlled, manipulated, threatened, and even stalked by their abusers.

> I thought being here [in jail] would keep me safe, at last. But no, he is still controlling me. He gets on the phone and won't let me talk with my sister who is trying to help me reach my lawyer. He refuses to bring my kids to see me, and tells them all kinds of things about me. He has threatened to hurt my mom if I say anything in court about him. I'll never make it out of here. I am totally alone here. . .isolated from my people when I need them most. It's like a double prison. (40-year-old woman detained in protective custody)
>
> Even these guards can't protect me. Do you know he had the nerve to push me against the wall and twist my arm way behind my back during a visit? It hurt so much! That was the arm he broke last year. They saw him, too, but no one helped. He just won't let up. He threatened to kill me once, and now I wonder if he'll do it while I am in here! (25-year-old woman serving two years in state prison)
>
> My kids have told me that he is messing with them [sexually abusing them] while I am gone. It made me sick, but at first I was afraid to tell because he said

he'd really take them if I report him. Well, I did anyways. And I hear nothing has been done. I just hope I get home soon because even though he beats me, that's better than him messing with my babies. I can't talk to anyone here about it because it would get me in trouble for not looking out for them. So I just got to beat my case [win my case] and hurry home to the madness. (31-year-old woman detained in urban jail)

As these accounts indicate, women continue to be as vulnerable to abuse as they were when they were arrested, and they may be returning to abusive relationships or high-risk environments. This situation is complicated by the nature of the community-based service delivery system that categorically offers services to "victims" without addressing the extent to which they are involved as "offenders" in illegal activities. This poses a serious barrier to services for women who cannot access services provided by anti-violence programs because of their illegal activity. There are disturbing accounts of such from victim advocates across the country whose funding will not allow them to serve women with an arrest record. The examples of institutional barriers to service permeate my research findings and point to the systemic nature of barriers to reintegration.

## Educational and Employment Services

The interviews revealed how significantly illegal activity and the circumstances that surround it interrupt educational and legal income-generating opportunities for many women. As reflected by the overall demographic profile of incarcerated women, few women I interviewed had steady employment, attended school, or had access to the training necessary to get a job at the time of their arrest (or the years leading up to it).

> I finished fifth grade. That's it. I couldn't go to school because of taking care of my brothers, and then I had to take care of my mom when she got sick. I liked school, but there was just too much else to do at home. Then it got to be too late because no school is going to take a 21-year-old in the fifth grade. I just lost my chance to make anything of myself. So I got involved in making money the only way I knew how. Living the life [street hustling]. I really do want to finish school though. (19-year-old woman detained in urban jail)
>
> For me, school was always hard. I never really learned to read, and I sure can't spell. All I can do is talk a good game. There was no kind of after-school program or place to help people like me. You at least need to know how to read to even find the reading programs! (28-year-old woman serving 12 years in state prison)
>
> I am 35 years old and have never had a legit [legitimate] job. No one taught me how to do an application, how to get dressed and show up, how to get

someone to hire me. Now that I have this X on my back [a criminal record] I'll never find someone to pay me. Not for a legit job anyways. (35-year-old-woman detained in a secured drug treatment program)

Although some of the women I interviewed held jobs or went to school during their incarceration, most prison- and jail-based rehabilitation programs have not been systematically evaluated, and most women report not having the academic or job-related skills or experience to support themselves once they are released.[24] They frequently depend on family members who themselves have limited resources, public agencies that have rigid eligibility requirements for their services, and/or episodic support from community-based agencies such as food pantries. The women I interviewed described how the pull toward illegal activity becomes stronger as they exhaust these options. Their accounts clearly establish the need for comprehensive educational, occupational, and income-generating opportunities when they are released from jails and prison.

When I leave here, I'm going to my mom's house. Me and everyone else. My uncle lives there with his old lady [female partner] and so does my two brothers and five sisters. No one has a job. There must be 20 people trying to eat off of her little check, and it just can't make it. Sometimes someone brings in something they got off the streets, but mostly the ones who get up early get to eat. Trouble is, they are over me now, so I don't know how long I can stay there. But the only other place I know to go is back to the crack house. No homeless shelter will take me, and I don't have any ID [identification] for public aid. I just hope there's room for me at my mom's or else I'll be right back here in general pop [general population at the jail]. (22-year-old woman detained in urban jail)

### Safe, Secure, Affordable Housing

As the previous account indicates, the women I interviewed described how the need for income and educational opportunities is closely related to the need for a place to live that is safe, secure, and affordable. Many incarcerated women have experienced repeated periods of homelessness. Most have families that are already overburdened, and in many cases their ties with their families have been severed as a result of their illegal activity. In my sample, all had been homeless at least once in their lives for three months or more, and all had lived most of their lives in overcrowded, substandard conditions. When they are released from jail or prison, they may be among the few fortunate women who have access to a transitional program or a treatment facility. However, these are typically only temporary arrangements, and most women are ultimately left on their own to find and secure long-term housing that they can afford. In my discussions with women being released from jail or prison, this is a constant worry.

> I am really scared and I need help badly. I just don't have anywhere to go that will help me avoid the people, places and things that brought me here in the first place. It is why that revolving door thing [arrest, release, rearrest] keeps spinning around and around. I am going right back out to the streets that lead me here. If only I had a place to go or a program close by that could help me get settled so that I could keep straight! (31-year-old woman detained in urban jail)

Regrettably, there are few community-based programs that address this need, and publicly funded low-income housing options are rapidly disappearing for women with criminal records, which creates yet another formidable systemic barrier.

## Child Advocacy and Family Reunification

One of the most compelling concerns that the women I interviewed described is the health and well-being of their children while they are separated from them.

> There is nothing more painful to a mother than to worry where her kids are while she is at the county [jail]. I worry day and night, and I just pray that wherever they are, they are being taken care of. If only someone would tell me where they are! For all I know, they are alone at home. When I got busted, I didn't even get to see them, and even though I sell drugs, I work hard to keep my babies off of the streets. I might lose them now, and if I do, I would do anything to get my kids back. The pain in my heart from worry is about to break me. (30-year-old woman detained in a secured drug treatment program)
>
> I'll do just about anything to myself, but don't let anyone come near my children. I love them as much as any mother . . . maybe even more since they suffer so much because of our situation. I have sacrificed, tried to give them what they need, and keep them as safe as I could. That's even when I was hungry, high or hurting from having been beaten. They always come first, and lots of what I did I thought I was doing to protect them. But it's hard to protect your babies when no one is protecting you. (22-year-old woman serving four years in state prison)

As these accounts illustrate, even in those instances where the nature of the illegal activity and the situations that women found themselves in created a less than optimal environment for child rearing, most women report worrying about their children both before and after they are arrested. The challenges of maintaining a relationship with children and other family members during periods of confinement are considerable, complicated by limited opportunities to visit, financial hardship, and emotional distress associated with the stigma of having a family member in jail.[25] There is considerable evidence that children of incarcerated mothers suffer emotionally, financially, and socially, yet there are few programs established to respond to this suffering.[26]

> If you think it's bad for me, imagine what me being in jail is like for my kids. Yes, they have suffered alright. They have no one to help them along now that I am here. No mother, no father, all of their friends make fun of them, and they don't have anyone in the world. At least if the judge is going to keep me here, he should give something for my kids. I worry that my boys are already headed down the wrong path because I'm not there to be watching out for them. Can't someone help my children? (27-year-old woman detained in urban jail)

Most women note that their children's suffering continues after their mother is released, and the issues related to custody of children, repairing relationships, parenting, and family reunification and stabilization are urgent and stressful.[27] Often the legal, practical, and emotional challenges are so overwhelming that women and their children never resolve the damage caused by the ruptured relationships.[28,29] Most of the women I have interviewed have lost at least one of their children to child protective services or the child welfare agency in her state. It should be emphasized that even if regaining custody is not a desirable option, the availability of services to assist in responding to these issues is critical to successful reintegration. My findings confirmed that when women are offered adequate support for being a parent, having even a non-custodial relationship with their children can be an important stabilizing force in women's lives as they make difficult transitions.

> I've been in and out of the joint [prison] for six years now. I've tried and tried and broken more promises that I thought was possible. I've lost friends, family, money, health, and my position in my community as a responsible citizen. And then, I got a second chance to raise my kids. When I was pregnant the last time and I got into a program, the world changed for me. It's hard to describe, but basically it is because of this five-month-old baby boy that I am clean, surviving one day at a time, and that I have hope for the future. I may never get to raise him on my own, but he is my reason for living. Who would have ever thought a baby could do such a thing? (31-year-old woman living in a recovery home)

## THE BROADER SOCIAL AND INSTITUTIONAL ANALYSIS

The challenges discussed in the previous section of this chapter must be understood within the broad social and institutional contexts of life for low-income women of color in disenfranchised neighborhoods. This section will discuss these contexts, as gleaned from the analysis of the data, as a way of conducting a meta-analysis of incarcerated women's needs. Three themes construct this broader context: (a) the impact of competing demands; (b) the need for institutional/community connections; and (c) the relevance of gender-specific and culturally-specific intervention. Consideration of these themes is necessary to create a deeper, more nuanced understanding of women returning from jail or prison. For, whereas the challenges reported during the interviews seem to fall into discrete issue areas, when the women describe them in their own words they become profoundly interrelated, and the ways that their lives are influenced by broader social forces become clear.

### The Impact of Competing Demands

The challenges women who are returning to their communities from jail or prison face are more complicated than the list of service needs would suggest. In fact, the demands and needs form a complex web of concerns and stressors that often compete with and exacerbate one another. The women I interviewed describe the co-occurrence of multiple demands as one of the most profound challenges they face when they are first released; this is a time characterized by fear, apprehension, lack of information about resources, and limited access to social support, as well as the more obvious emotions, such as relief.

The impact of these multiple and competing demands is illustrated by this example of a typical woman who may be simultaneously attempting to regain custody of her children, looking for an apartment and a job, and trying to get into a substance abuse treatment program as a condition of her probation or parole.

> I start my day running to drop my urine [drug testing]. Then I go see my children, show up for my training program, look for a job, go to a meeting [Alcoholics Anonymous] and show up at my part-time job. I have to take the bus everywhere, sometimes eight buses for four hours a day. I don't have the proper outer clothes, I don't have money to buy lunch along the way, and everyone who works with me keeps me waiting so that I am late to my next appointment. If I fail any one of these things and my PO [probation officer] finds out, I am revoked [probation is revoked]. I am so tired that I sometimes fall asleep on my way home from work at 2 a.m. and that's dangerous given where I live. And then the next day, I have to start over again. I don't mind being busy and working hard . . . that's part of my recovery. But this is a situation that is setting me

> up to fail. I just can't keep up and I don't know where to start. I want my kids. I need a place to stay. I have to have a job, meetings to keep me clean, and I am required to be in job training. (26-year-old woman living with grandmother)

The women in this sample described how the demands of any one of these urgent needs might consume most of their material and emotional resources. As the previous account suggests, the combination of the competing demands may seriously interfere with successful reintegration: the woman will need an apartment to regain custody of her children, she will need a job to get an apartment, she will need to get treatment for her addiction to be able to work, and initial contact with her children may only be possible during business hours if they are in custody of the state. The demands multiply and compound each other, and services are typically offered by agencies in different locations. Competing needs without any social support to meet them may seriously limit a woman's chances for success in the challenging process of reintegration.

### Institutional/Community Connection

As previously noted, most of the women incarcerated in jails and prisons in the US come from and return to disenfranchised communities with limited economic, social, and political resources. The women I interviewed were no different. They describe in considerable detail how the experiences and circumstances that have been difficult for them (such as lack of affordable housing, joblessness, domestic violence, and limited health care) and that led to illegal activity will most likely not have changed. In fact, many of the women I interviewed anticipate that these conditions may become worse. Experiences have shown them that services will probably not be readily available to their families. They believe public policy decisions to divest from low-income communities and reduce support programs in marginalized poor areas have had a serious negative impact on life for many citizens, and they can point to specific examples of such. When coupled with the criminal justice policies that have led to the growing rates of incarceration of residents from their low-income communities, the individual and collective impact has been disastrous.[3] The future of public housing is bleak, the opportunities for public assistance are increasingly limited, the availability of legal assistance has been seriously curtailed, and changes in Medicaid and managed health care result in limited access to health and mental health services. Women with criminal records who are facing the competing demands previously described are arguably in one of the worst positions to secure the services they need, both because the communities' resources are so seriously limited and because their criminal record further inhibits their access to services.

Do you know what it is like to try to get through the day with an X on your back [a criminal record]? People don't want to hire you, no one wants to rent you an apartment, you can't count on your family because they have given up on you, your church calls you a sinner, and no one trusts you. I've done my time. But coming home is like having to do time again in your own community where folks just won't forgive you or lend you a helping hand. (29-year-old woman living with friends)

From their perspective, this situation is complicated further by the reduction in services offered inside correctional facilities in the US. Several recent reports indicate that jails and prisons are offering fewer educational programs, fewer comprehensive treatment services, and generally more limited opportunities for counseling, discharge planning, and rehabilitation. Similar to the worsening conditions in the communities where they live, women describe the conditions in correctional facilities as harsher; their sentences are longer and served in more isolated rural areas where there are fewer rehabilitation programs available to them. An analysis that incorporates this understanding of the institutional/ community connection argues for neighborhood development efforts so that women who are released find their community equipped to provide the support that they need.

### Gender-Specific and Culturally Sensitive Needs

Analysis of the data from the interviews conducted for this chapter revealed important insights into the ways that gender, ethnic identity, and economic status converge to make the situation incarcerated women face very complicated. It could be argued that many of the needs and dynamics that the women reported in this study affect the men as well as the women in the communities. Most of the current research, however, points to the ways that participation in illegal activities and the experience of incarceration is different for women and men. As such, the challenges that influence successful reintegration are decidedly gendered, and cultural issues play a significant role in successful engagement and program retention.[13,30,31] For instance, it is suggested that parenting classes that are taught by women from the same cultural and economic background as the "students" are most helpful.[32] In this and other ways, attention to cultural and gender identity, as broad influences on both behavior and opportunity, must be incorporated into an understanding of what women being released from jails and prisons need to successfully reintegrate in their racial/ethnic communities upon release from jail or prison.

It's like we are all used to the brothers [men] getting locked up. But no one has any sympathy for us when we go down [go to prison]. It's like we are somehow supposed to not get caught up [involved in illegal activity] the way they do. But it is getting just as bad . . . no it is worse for us now. There is no way to make it without running the streets to support yourself. Plus, the cops are now looking more for women than for the brothers. It's like they are after us now. And they get us good! But folks don't realize that. (38-year-old woman detained in urban jail)

This situation is reflected in the sentiment on the part of some incarcerated women I interviewed who felt that their needs as women are not a priority in their disenfranchised communities.

There's a lot of pressure in my neighborhood and not enough programs to go around. I guess on the one hand I understand it, but on the other hand, I think I deserve as much attention as the other folks around here. They take care of the seniors . . . well they aren't all so nice, and they watch out for the kids who are beaten by the cops . . . well lots of them did things wrong. Even the bums on the street are treated better than women who come home. It's like we get only what is left over from all of the other people who need things . . . the sick and shut in, the people with AIDS, the abandoned babies . . . there just isn't enough programs to go around. (42-year-old woman living with her children in a homeless shelter)

Women of color returning from jail or prison do not feel embraced by their communities, and they are not identified as having the right to demand services from it. The sense of being marginalized within the context of a disenfranchised community has a profound impact on the ability of women to successfully reintegrate into it. A deeper analysis of this issue is needed to identify elements of gender-specific and culturally sensitive approaches to this work.

## WHAT WORKS: FOUR APPROACHES

While identifying the individual challenges and systemic barriers women face when they return to their communities from jail or prison, evidence of the conditions that might facilitate the process of reintegration emerged. In this section, I will discuss four key elements of programmatic and neighborhood improvement, emphasizing the notion that women not only need more comprehensive services but that economic conditions in their neighborhoods need to change for them to successfully reengage with community life.

## Comprehensive Programs

At the programmatic level, women need programs that are comprehensive and that offer what have been called "wraparound services."[33] In these approaches, women who are returning to their communities are able to get assistance with multiple needs in one place; the intervention plans take into account the multiple demands they may be addressing simultaneously. This type of intervention is often referred to in the literature as a "case management approach" and has been credited with important enhancements over more traditional strategies for working with women in need.[34,35] In general, these types of programs offer a more holistic approach that incorporates the gender-specific and culturally specific needs comprehensively.

## Community Development and Linkages

Concomitant with concrete services that help women reintegrate into their communities upon release from jails or prisons, successful programs also focus on strengthening the community's capacity to work with this population. Community-based organizations need to build linkages with other services, and they need to be involved in programs that are designed to prevent incarceration in the first place. Because most people seek services close to where they live, such an approach would mean more coordination at the neighborhood level, and it would emphasize strengthening organizational capacity to meet the needs that are described earlier in this chapter. This strategy would necessitate providing services that are culturally appropriate and consistent with what women in the community need, and it would require agencies to work with women who are incarcerated in correctional facilities prior to their release to the community. A community-development approach would incorporate policy-level work, community organizing, and social-change strategies to increase the quality of community life overall and for women specifically.

## Empowerment or Consciousness-Raising Approach

Social science literature has only recently looked at different theoretical orientations to working with populations of vulnerable women. A consciousness-raising or empowerment approach, based on the work of Paulo Freire,[36] suggests that a key influence on a person's ability to make individual change is the extent to which he or she has an understanding of the multiple influences on his or her behavior. This approach has been used in work with battered women, women living in public housing, adolescent girls in reducing the risk of youth violence, and women facing serious health risks.[37] As applied to women involved in illegal activities, an empowerment approach facilitates an intervention process that is based on strategies to help women develop critical insight into the structural influences on their personal choices (as opposed to approaches that foster self-blame or focus only on issues such as self-esteem). Instead, this approach focuses on enhancing women's decision-making skills within the context of limited options and involving women as key social actors in expanding the options they have.

In addition, empowerment and consciousness-raising programs allow formerly incarcerated women to reject some of the social stigmas they face by becoming members of self-help networks in their communities. Those programs that use this approach describe women's success as being linked to their ability to shift their point of view from self-blame to self-responsibility and ultimately to responsibility for one's family and neighborhood. Developing a sense of hope, an orientation toward the future, and the willingness to take responsibility are identified as objectives on which success of these programs would be measured. Programmatic approaches that incorporate such an approach are particularly important given the feelings of inevitability and hopelessness that are reported to characterize the experiences of women who are most frequently arrested in the US.

### Community Mentoring, Care, and Consistency

Finally, there is a set of structural characteristics of programs and neighborhoods that enhances the successful reintegration of women from jails and prisons into their communities.[38] These conditions center around how the women are perceived by neighbors and program staff, and the extent to which the community and the programs have the resources (and the will) to meet women's needs. The first element that seems critical to this approach is linked to program staffing. Most services that are successful in helping women reintegrate into the community have hired (or are otherwise influenced by) women who have been similarly situated. The extent to which women have a peer and/or mentoring relationship with someone whom they perceive is "like them" is critical. This element – being able to identify and learn from successful role models and mentors from one's own neighborhood – is key.

The second set of features that are essential for women being released back to their communities from correctional facilities includes stability and predictability. Consistent activities that are structured around what women need, adequate resources for long-term support, and opportunities to work collectively and to develop a sense of community all seem to facilitate reentry. Some literature argues that residential programs are most successful, others suggest small store-front operations in the community work best, whereas others still advocate for restorative justice programs. In any of these cases, the critical elements are that women are engaged as partners in reentry and that their needs are placed in the center of community-development initiatives.

## CONCLUSION

Research conducted on the concrete challenges women being released from jail and prison experience and an analysis of the broader issues they face in the community point to the urgent need for social reform. The nature of the reform centers on both enhanced service delivery and systematic change in low-income communities of color from which the majority of the incarcerated female population in the US is drawn. When they are released, women need comprehensive programs, better treatment, wraparound services, empowerment programs, and opportunities for self-sufficiency. Discharge planning programs, ex-offender peer group support, mother-child programs, and intermediate sanctions all emerged as potential programmatic initiatives. These programs need to be evaluated and replicated in various communities, and more longitudinal research needs to be conducted to evaluate the impact of women's incarceration on individual and community life.

In addition, the analysis of the interviews reviewed in this chapter indicated that beyond expanded services, women need community conditions to change for them to return successfully to their communities and avoid rearrest. They need families that are not divided by public policy, streets and homes that are safe from violence and abuse, and health and mental health services that are accessible. The challenges women face must be met with expanded opportunity and a more thoughtful criminal justice policy. This would require a plan for reinvestment in low-income communities that centers around women's need for safety and self-sufficiency. If undertaken, such a reform agenda might even prevent some of the arrests and incarcerations of women from low-income communities in the first place.

## REFERENCES

1 Bureau of Justice Statistics. *Women Offenders: special report*. Washington, DC: US Department of Justice; 1999.

2 Bureau of Justice Statistics. *Criminal Offenders Statistics*. Washington, DC: US Department of Justice; 2000.

3 Mauer M, Potler C, Wolf R. *Gender and Justice: women, drugs and sentencing policy*. Washington, DC: The Sentencing Project; 1999.

4 Freudenberg N, Wilets I, Greene MB, *et al*. Linking women in jail to community services: factors associated with rearrest and retention of drug-using women following release from jail. *J Am Med Womens Assoc*. 1998; **53**(2): 89–93.

5 US Department of Housing and Urban Development. *State of the Cities – 1999*. Washington, DC: Government Printing Office; 1999.

6 Browne A, Miller B, Maguin E. Prevalence and severity of lifetime physical and sexual victimization among incarcerated women. *Int J Law Psychiatry*. 1999; **22**(3–4): 301–22.

7 Richie BE. *Compelled to Crime: the gender entrapment of battered black women*. New York, NY: Routledge; 1996.

8 Blank S, McDonnell DD, Rubin SR, *et al*. New approaches to syphilis control. Finding opportunities for syphilis treatment and congenital syphilis prevention in a women's correctional setting. *Sex Transm Dis*. 1997; **24**(4): 218–26.

9 Bond L, Semaan S. At risk for HIV infection: incarcerated women in a county jail in Philadelphia. *Women and Health*. 1996; **24**(4): 27–45.

10 Hammett TM, Gaiter JL, Crawford C. Reaching seriously at-risk populations: health interventions in criminal justice settings. *Health Educ Behav*. 1998; **25**(1): 99–120.

11 Waterston A. *Street Addicts in the Political Economy*. Philadelphia, PA: Temple University Press; 1993.

12 Henderson DJ. Drug abuse and incarcerated women: a research review. *J Subst Abuse Treat*. 1998; **15**(6): 579–87.

13 Morash M, Bynum TS, Koons BA. *Women Offenders: programming needs and promising approaches*. Washington, DC: National Institute of Justice; 1998.

14 Prendergast M, Wellish J, Falkin GP. Assessment of and services for substance-abusing women offenders in community and correctional settings. *Prison J*. 1995; **75**: 240–56.

15 Taylor SD. Women offenders and reentry issues. *J Psychoactive Drugs*. 1996; **28**(1): 85–93.

16 Reinarman C, Levine HG. *Crack in America: demon drugs and social justice*. Berkeley, CA: University of California Press; 1998.

17 Belknap J. Access to programs and health care for incarcerated women. *Federal Probation*. 1996; **LX**(4): 34–9.

18 Richie BE, Johnsen C. Abuse histories among newly incarcerated women in a New York City jail. *J Am Med Womens Assoc*. 1996; **51**(3): 111–14, 117.

19 Broome KM, Knight K, Hiller ML, *et al*. Drug treatment process indicators for probationers and prediction of recidivism. *J Subst Abuse Treat*. 1996; **13**(6): 487–91.

20 Hammett TM, Harmon P, Maruschak LM. *1996–1997 Update: HIV/AIDS, STDs, and TB in Correctional Facilities*. Washington, DC: US Department of Justice; 1999.

21 Steadman HE, Veysey BM. Providing services for jail inmates with mental disorders. In: *National Institute of Justice Research: In Brief* (US Department of Justice Publication No. NCJ 162207). Washington, DC: US Department of Justice; 1997.

22 Teplin LA, Abram KM, McClelland GM. Prevalence of psychiatric disorders among incarcerated women. I. Pretrial jail detainees. *Arch Gen Psychiatry*. 1996; **53**(6): 505–12.

23 Bill L. The victimization . . . and . . . revictimization of female offenders. *Corrections Today*. 1998; **60**: 106–11.

24 Koons B, Burrow JD, Morash M, *et al*. Expert and offender perceptions of program elements linked to successful outcomes for incarcerated women. *Crime Delinq*. 1997; **43**(4): 512–32.

25 Katz P. Supporting families and children of mothers in jail: an integrated child welfare and criminal justice strategy. *Child Welfare*. 1998; **77**: 495–511.

26 Blakeley S. California program to focus on new mothers. *Corrections Today*. 1995; **57**(7): 128–30.

27 Morton J, Williams D. Mother/child bonding: incarcerated women struggle to maintain meaningful relationships with their children. *Corrections Today*. 1998; **60**(7): 98–105.

28 DeGroot G. A day in the life: four women share their stories of life behind bars. *Corrections Today.* 1998; **60**(7): 82–6, 96.

29 Dressel P, Porterfield J, Barnhill SK. Mothers behind bars. *Corrections Today.* 1998; **60**: 90–4.

30 Miller B. Different, not more difficult: gender-specific training helps bridge the gap. *Corrections Today.* 1998; **60**: 142–4.

31 Morris A, Wilkinson C. Responding to female prisoners' needs. *Prison J.* 1995; **75**(3): 295–305.

32 Schaffner L. Families on probation: court-ordered parenting skills classes for parents of juvenile offenders. *Crime Delinq.* 1997; **43**: 412–37.

33 Reed BG. Drug misuse and dependency in women: the meaning and implications of being considered a special population or minority group. *International Journal of Addictions.* 1985; **20**(1): 13–62.

34 Martin SS, Inciardi JA. Case management approaches for the criminal justice client in drug treatment and criminal justice. In: Inciardi JA, editor. *Criminal Justice.* Thousand Oaks, CA: Sage Publications; 1993.

35 Rhodes W, Gross M. *Case Management Reduces Drug Use and Criminality among Drug-involved Arrestees: an experimental study of an HIV prevention intervention.* Washington, DC: National Institute of Justice and National Institute of Drug Abuse; 1997.

36 Freire P. *Pedagogy of the Oppressed,* translated by Myra Bergman Ramos. New York, NY: Continuum Publishing Company; 1998/1970.

37 Wallerstein N. Powerlessness, empowerment, and health: implications for health promotion. *Am J Health Promot.* 1992; **6**(3): 197–205.

38 Vigilante KC, Flynn MM, Affleck PC, *et al.* Reduction in recidivism of incarcerated women through primary care, peer counseling, and discharge planning. *J Womens Health.* 1999; **8**(3): 409–15.

# CHAPTER 4

# Women, Health and Prisons in Australia

Judy Parker, Debbie Kilroy and Jonathan Hirst

In the Western world the prison epitomizes the custodial power of the state in relation to control and punishment. It is argued here that the modern criminal justice system is primarily concerned with punishment and containment and there appears to be little place to address physical, mental and psychosocial health concerns. In Australia, incarceration rates vary by state and territory, but all show that indigenous women are incarcerated at a rate higher than any other group, that there has been an increase in women imprisoned for robbery related to drug use, and that rates of mental disorder among women in prison appear to be higher than those in the general community.

This chapter draws upon relevant data to examine the physical, mental and psychosocial characteristics of women in Australian prisons as well as the economic and social circumstances that contributed to their incarceration. These characteristics and circumstances suggest a need for greater emphasis on care, treatment and rehabilitation within prisons and raise questions about the appropriateness of prison for women in many cases. The chapter discusses: (a) patterns of women's incarceration and their drug use; (b) women within forensic mental health services; and (c) Aboriginal and Torres Strait Islander women within the criminal justice system. Our purpose is to demonstrate the health difficulties they experience and to argue the importance of a shift from the prison-based to community-based care with provision of adequate social and health services.

Australia's eight states and territories each have their own public health system, health legislation, criminal codes and correctional services. Data relating to women in prison are not necessarily collected in uniform ways and are gathered from a number of sources. Prisoners counted in the National Prisoner Census of 2002 included 1484 women, which comprised 6.6% of the total prison population and 0.0076% of the total Australian population.[1] More recently, in the quarter to March 2008, 1853 of the average daily number of full-time prisoners were women, which comprised 7% of the total prison population.[2] The percentage of women prisoners in Australia is comparable to the US and slightly higher than in England and Wales (5.6%), and New Zealand and Canada, which are both around 5%.[1]

The Australian Institute of Criminology (AIC) has brought together data from police annual reports in the three jurisdictions that release such data, the national police custody survey, and the Drug Use Monitoring in Australia program.[3] The number of women incarcerated in Australian prisons nearly doubled between 1991 and 2001.[4] The most recent AIC figures, in 2006, indicate a 5% increase in women in prison over the previous year.[3]

Increasingly it is recognized that co-morbid substance use and mental health disorders are the expectation rather than the exception within the Australian female prison population. Very high proportions of women prisoners test positive to exposure to hepatitis C[5] and a higher proportion of women prisoners report chronic physical conditions (particularly asthma) than women in the general population.[1] They are also more likely than women in the general population to have a history characterized by experiences of physical and/or sexual abuse, childhood trauma, exposure to domestic violence, poverty and social deprivation.[6] The patterns of incarceration for Aboriginal and Torres Strait Islander women are so concerning that their specific situation is addressed separately later in this chapter.

## WOMEN'S INCARCERATION AND DRUG USE

Women's drug use appears to be a defining factor in their participation in crime, although drawing an inference of direct causality between drug use and offending behavior by women is overly simplistic. While a number of interventions have been implemented with the aim of reducing reoffending, the factors underlying both drug use and crime need to be taken into account in holistically designed and integrated programs for persons with drug use disorders. Drug and alcohol counseling and methadone programs have been used in a number of correctional settings with some success,[7] but are likely to be limited in their effectiveness if they are not supported by interventions that address a range of critical factors. These factors include underlying mental health concerns, poor education, weak social and emotional skills, poverty, and limited support systems which are frequently found to coexist and interact with drug use disorders.[8]

A survey of women in Queensland prisons[9] found that 95% had experienced childhood abuse (physical and sexual) at the hands of family members, which was seen as a contributing factor in their drug use. Although prison was a negative experience for women in the study, it was particularly difficult for those who continued to self-medicate, share needles, and engage in other self-harm behaviors. In another study in New South Wales, prisoners reported that methadone programs were not effective as a sole intervention, due to the failure to explore and treat the underlying reasons for drug dependence.[10]

As Cameron[4] notes, while drug intervention programs can be important, their effect is limited when effort is not also put into encouraging women to be self supporting through education and employment programs. More holistic drug use intervention programs that focus on a wider therapeutic framework are currently provided to Victorian women prisoners by the psychological services provider, Caranich.[4]

One program that has sought to keep people out of prison and shows promising results to date is the drug court.[11] This program set up in New South Wales diverts women from prison and into treatment emphasizing social support and development of living skills. The program includes regular reports to the courts, and urine testing. Over the duration of the one-year program, participants are expected to stabilize their lives as they develop life and job skills. Drug and alcohol counseling in such community-based programs appears to be more effective as the complex social needs of the women prisoners can be met and supports can be developed outside the antisocial and demoralizing environment of prisons. Of course the success of such programs is limited by the availability of resources provided in the community.

Prison is a costly and inefficient means of containment of women whose offending is predominantly or significantly linked to substance misuse. Given the increasing number of women being incarcerated for drug-related crimes, clearly the deterrent effect of a punitive approach is ineffective. While this approach pervades the corrections systems of Australia, efforts to provide drug and alcohol counseling utilizing motivational interviewing, empathy, and unconditional positive regard are significantly undermined.

There is an urgent need for community-based care for women convicted of drug-related offenses, where they can be provided with refuge and support to heal and get on with their lives. Community support is the crucial key. At present there appears to be little political will to provide sustained and sustaining support for women caught in the cycle of drug use and imprisonment with all the devastating consequences upon their health, their relationships, their families, and their communities.

## WOMEN AND FORENSIC MENTAL HEALTH SERVICES

In Australia, there is an assumption that persons with mental illness who become involved in the criminal justice system are the responsibility of forensic mental health services. Some argue that until recently forensic mental health services remained invisible to the general community "except at moments of scandal."[12(p.435)] However, some states have developed modern systems which focus on therapeutic as well as assessment services. A code, promulgated in 1995 with the aim of serving as a prototype for all Australian jurisdictions, includes the new defense of mental impairment, which has been adopted, albeit with modifications, within most jurisdictions.[12] A finding of mental impairment, or of unfitness to plead, is in most cases decided by the court and results in detention in a hospital or release into the community. When people with mental illness are convicted, they may be ordered by the court to undergo psychiatric treatment in a hospital or in the community.

Because the provision of forensic mental health services is the responsibility of state and territory governments, each with their own mental health legislation, service models can differ substantially. "In New South Wales, the most populous state, the bulk of that state's forensic public mental health inpatient services are [sic] provided by the hospital of a correctional facility, Long Bay Prison, whereas, in contrast, Victoria centers its services in a recently built 120 bed stand alone mental health facility."[12(p.438)]

In several jurisdictions, the old psychiatric hospitals have been closed down and services have shifted to the community. This move has resulted in a limited capacity for the containment and care of "difficult" patients, and experts have called for increased forensic mental health services. Women suffering from mental disorders, who are not dangerous to others, could be diverted away from the criminal justice system to appropriate community-based mental health settings. However, such services are patchily distributed within Australia.

One Victorian organization known as Forensicare offers court, prison, hospital and community-based services and receives referrals from the courts, general mental health services, police, prisons and justice agencies.[10] Within Forensicare, the Thomas Embling Hospital has a national and possibly an international reputation as a dedicated forensic psychiatric hospital of 100 beds.[12] The women's care program there is unique in Australia and one of only a few around the world. However, the beds available are not sufficient to meet the need.

In a risk-averse society such as Australia, preoccupation with danger assessment often leads to control and containment approaches to behavioral problems rather than supportive management. This societal mindset encourages a view of people with mental disorders based on their supposed level of dangerousness. With the current shortage of dedicated hospital beds for people suffering acute episodes of mental illness, women who behave inappropriately due to severe symptoms of a psychiatric illness can find themselves in prison when they would be treated more effectively within a safe, community environment. Many of these women do not present a serious threat to others; therefore, questions of social justice have to be raised about their presence within a prison environment.

Three recent successful appeals to the Victorian Supreme Court highlight that the judiciary has at least in part accepted that the prison environment is unable to provide vulnerable women with the therapeutic mental health services necessary for successful rehabilitation. In *R v Wooden* [2006] VSCA 97, *R v SH* [2006] VSCA 83, and *R v Rollo* [2006] VSCA 154,[13] the court reduced the sentences of women prisoners due to the deterioration of their psychiatric conditions while in prison.

## ABORIGINAL AND TORRES STRAIT ISLANDER WOMEN WITHIN THE CRIMINAL JUSTICE SYSTEM

Indigenous Australians represent approximately 2% of the total Australian population. Their life expectancy is approximately 17 years less than that of the non-indigenous population. In 2003–4, in all age groups below 65, the age-specific death rates for Aboriginal and Torres Strait Islander Australians were at least twice those experienced by the non-indigenous population. Infant mortality was three times that of non-indigenous infants. Hospitalization for ischemic heart disease among Aboriginal and Torres Strait Islander women was four times the rate of the general population. Rates of communicable diseases were higher and oral health was reported as poor. Over one-third of Aboriginal and Torres Strait Islander people 15 years or older reported a disability or long-term health problem. They were twice as likely to be hospitalized for psychological and behavioral disorders. Hospitalization rates for assault and self-harm were seven times more likely among men and 31 times more likely among women than in the general population.[14]

Indigenous women are currently incarcerated at a rate higher than any other group in Australia.[4] While the incarceration rate for women from 1991–2001 increased by 147%, the rate of increase of indigenous women was 255.8%. In March 2004, indigenous women were imprisoned nationally at a rate 20.8 times that of non-indigenous women.[1] Although incarceration rates vary by state, all show over-representation by indigenous women. In Western Australia in the period July 1, 2001 to June 30, 2002, indigenous women constituted 51.7% of all women received into prison despite constituting 3.2% of the female population of Western Australia. Recidivism rates are very high among indigenous women, with national statistics showing that three-quarters of all indigenous female prisoners have been previously imprisoned.[15]

A significant factor in the incarceration of indigenous women is fine defaulting in relation to public order offenses such as public drunkenness and swearing in public. These women are incarcerated because the burden of paying fines is very difficult for them. That they receive shorter sentences compared with non-indigenous women suggests that indigenous women are not being provided with non-custodial sentencing options that are available to non-indigenous women.

A report by the Anti-Discrimination Commission in Queensland[16] noted that indigenous women **are particularly at risk of discrimination in prison.** The prison system does not adequately attend to their unique needs despite providing a wide range of programs that address the specific needs of female indigenous prisoners.

The Social Justice Report by the Aboriginal and Torres Strait Islander Social Justice Commissioner[15] noted:

> The rising rate of over-representation of indigenous women is occurring in the context of intolerably high levels of family violence, over-policing for selected offences, unemployment and poverty. Studies of indigenous women in prison reveal experiences of life in a society fraught with danger and violence. The consequences to the community of the removal of indigenous women are significant and potentially expose children to risk of neglect, abuse, hunger and homelessness.[15(p.2)]

This Report concluded that:

> The discrimination faced by Indigenous women is more than a combination of race, gender and class. It includes dispossession, cultural oppression, disrespect of spiritual beliefs, economic disempowerment, but from traditional economies, not just post-colonial economies and more. Non-discrimination includes more than an aspiration for standards identical to those of the dominant culture. It requires equal respect for difference.[15(p.155)]

The justice system of Australia has historically demonstrated duplicity in the treatment of Aboriginal women. While it has shown a readiness to punish Aboriginal women, it has not demonstrated a similar preparedness to protect them. In a key lecture on law and human rights, Professor Larissa Behrendt[17] commented on a case in which a judge reduced the sentences of the male perpetrators in a sexual assault on an indigenous woman. In spite of evidence to the contrary, the judge argued that sexual assault is not considered as serious in Aboriginal communities as it is in white communities. Professor Behrendt made the further point in her lecture that Australia's institutions of justice and correction entrench Aboriginal woman as both victims and offenders. She concluded that the creation of a culture in which Aboriginal women are disempowered, victimized and unprotected leaves them growing up seeing and experiencing violence and sexual abuse, and thinking of it as normal.

## SUMMARY

Within Australian society the female prison population has higher levels of mental illness, injecting drug use, experiences of trauma, violence and social disadvantage than the male prison population. However, the smaller number of women prisoners does not allow for the diverse range of therapeutic programs available to the male prison population. Rather than providing a therapeutic environment, the modern prison serves to isolate and segregate women. Stoller's[18] comments about the US prison environment are equally applicable in Australia:

> ... where medicine attempts to provide cure and management of disease, the primary goal of 21st century corrections (despite the implications of training and rehabilitation in the word correction) is typically detention and punishment.[18(p.2)]

While each of the jurisdictions within Australia has to varying degrees implemented programs aimed at improving the health problems of women prisoners, the effectiveness of most of these programs has not been evaluated. Any such evaluation is likely to discover that their aims to rehabilitate and reduce recidivism are undermined by a prison environment where punishment and containment remain primary.

For the health services of women's prisons at least to meet those in the community two possible scenarios can be envisaged. In the first, the governmental authorities would allocate significant resources to develop a holistic and integrated corrections system. Such a system would provide a range of facilities and programs specifically designed to meet women's health and rehabilitative needs. However, for this to be successful, a major culture change within the prison system would need to occur. In the second, recognition would be given to the mounting evidence that the prison environment exacerbates disadvantage and discrimination and facilitates the creation and maintenance of criminal behavior. Strategies would then need to be developed to implement community-based programs aimed at healing the wounds suffered by women who have been victims of an uncaring society. This is the hope for the future and any moves toward such an approach are to be welcomed.

## REFERENCES

1 Australian Bureau of Statistics. *Australian Social Trends: crime and justice: women in prison* (No. 4102.0). 2004. Available at: www.abs.gov.au/Ausstats/abs@.nsf/7d12b0 f6763c78caca257061001cc588/781c132ae9185bedca256e9e002975fc!OpenDocum ent (accessed July 2, 2008).
2 Australian Bureau of Statistics. *Summary of Findings: corrective services Australia March*

*quarter* (No. 4512.0). 2008. Available at: www.abs.gov.au/AUSSTATS/abs@.nsf/Pro ductsbyReleaseDate/9A15EFC4A9079005CA25746C001C0FD7?OpenDocument (accessed July 2, 2008).

3 Australian Institute of Criminology. *Crime and Criminal Justice Statistics: female prisoners.* Canberra: Australian Institute of Criminology; 2008. Available at: www.aic.gov. au/stats/cjs/corrections/females/ (accessed July 30, 2008).

4 Cameron M. *Women Prisoners and Correctional Programs. Trends and Issues in Crime and Criminal Justice, No. 194.* Canberra: Australian Institute of Criminology; 2001. Available at: www.hawaii.edu/hivandaids/Women%20Prisoners%20and%20 Correctional%20Programs.pdf (accessed July 28, 2008).

5 Ministerial Advisory Committee on AIDS, Sexual Health and Hepatitis C Sub-Committee. *Hepatitis C Virus Projections Working Group: estimates and projections of the Hepatitis C virus epidemic in Australia.* Darlinghurst, New South Wales: National Centre in HIV Epidemiology and Clinical Research; 2006. Available at: www. hepcawareness.net.au/PDFs/est&proj_report_06.pdf (accessed May 25, 2009).

6 Australian Senate Select Committee on Mental Health. *A National Approach to Mental Health – From Crisis to Community (First Report).* 2006. Available at: www.aph.gov.au/ Senate/committee/mentalhealth_ctte/report/c14.htm (accessed August 13, 2007).

7 Dolan KA, Shearer J, MacDonald M, *et al.* A randomized controlled trial of methadone maintenance treatment versus wait list control in an Australian prison system. *Drug Alcohol Depend.* 2003; **72**: 59–65.

8 Johnson H. *Drugs and Crime: a study of incarcerated female offenders.* Canberra: Australian Institute of Criminology; 2004. Available at: www.aic.gov.au/publications /rpp/63/RPP63.pdf (accessed May 25, 2009).

9 Kilroy D. *When will you see the real us? Women in prison.* 2000. Paper presented at Women in Corrections: Staff and Clients Conference convened by the Australian Institute of Criminology in conjunction with the Department of Correctional Services SA. Adelaide October 31–November 1, 2000.

10 Hampton B. *Prisons and Women: Victorian Institute of Forensic Mental Health annual report 2002/3.* Sydney: New South Wales University Press; 1993.

11 Freeman K, Karski RL, Doak P. New South Wales drug court evaluation: program and participant profiles. *C & J Bulletin.* 2000; 50. Available at: www.lawlink.nsw.gov. au/lawlink/bocsar/ll_bocsar.nsf/vwFiles/CJB50.pdf/$file/CJB50.pdf#target='_blank' (accessed May 25, 2009).

12 Mullen PE, Briggs S, Dalton T, *et al.* Forensic mental health services in Australia. *Int J Law Psychiatry.* 2000; **23**: 433–52.

13 Victorian Supreme Court of Australia *R v Rollo* [2006] VSCA 154 (Warren and Vincent, JJ); *R v SH* [2006] VSCA 83 (Warren, Charles and Chernov, JJ); *R v Wooden* [2006] VSCA 97 (Callaway and Vincent, JJ).

14 Human Rights and Equal Opportunity Commission. *A Statistical Overview of Aboriginal and Torres Strait Islander Peoples in Australia.* 2006. Available at: www.hreoc. gov.au/Social_Justice/statistics/index.html (accessed July 26, 2008).

15 Aboriginal and Torres Strait Islander Social Justice Commission. *Social Justice Report 2002.* Available at: www.hreoc.gov.au/social_Justice/sj_report/sjreport02/index.html (accessed May 25, 2009).

16 Anti-Discrimination Commission Queensland. *Women in Prison: a report by the Anti-*

*Discrimination Commission Queensland.* 2006. Available at: www.adcq.qld.gov.au/Project-WIP/WIPreport_6.5.htm (accessed July 26, 2008).

17 Behrendt L. *As good as it gets or as good as it could be? Benchmarking human rights in Australia.* Paper presented at the Freilich Foundation Alice Tay Memorial Lecture on Law and Human Rights. May 18, 2006. Old Canberra House, Australian National University. Available at: www.anu.edu.au/hrc/freilich/events/2006/AliceTay1%20lecture-behrendt.pdf (accessed July 2, 2008).

18 Stoller N. Space, place and movement as aspects of health care in three women's prisons. *Soc Sci Med.* 2003; **56**: 2263–75.

# CHAPTER 5

# Incarceration of Women in Britain: A Matter of Madness

## Paul Godin and Kathleen Kendall

Similar to other Anglophone countries, Britain has followed the US and imprisoned an ever larger proportion of its population. Though Britain's prison population is dwarfed by the mass incarceration of the US, Britain holds the unenviable claim to incarcerate a higher proportion of its population than any other European country. As in the US, this rise in incarceration in Britain has little association with the crime rate. Prison statistics are compiled differently in the various countries of Britain, making aggregation difficult. Therefore, those held for England and Wales, where the vast majority of people within Britain reside, are commonly used as a guide for the nation as a whole. Between 1989 and 1992 Britain experienced a 50% increase in its crime rate, yet at the same time the prison population of England and Wales fell from 50 000 to 42 000.[1] Thereafter, the crime rate increased less dramatically, though the prison population almost doubled and now stands at just under 80 000.[2]

This rise is largely associated with more crimes carrying a prison sentence than before, particularly drug-related crimes, and longer sentences for individuals appearing before the court. What the Home Office calls a policy of "more severe response to less serious offenses"[3(p.21)] has led to a significant increase in the imprisonment of women, whose crimes are generally less violent and less serious than those of men. Between 1991 and 2001, the number of women entering prison rose by 223%, compared with 74% for men.[4] The number of women in prison within England and Wales rose from 1560 in 1993 to 4672 in 2004, before dropping slightly to 4248 in 2006.[5] Such figures convey little about the human experiences of those who lie behind them. However, Women in Prison,[6] a charity that campaigns against the incarceration of women, reports the following shocking statistics about the deprivation, despair, and poor mental health of women in British prisons: (a) 20% have been cared for by the state away from their family as children; (b) 50% report being victims of childhood abuse or domestic violence; (c) 70% have mental health problems; (d) 37% have attempted suicide; and (e) 27 committed suicide in 2003/4. Leanne Gidney, an 18-year-old single parent found hanging in her cell after being jailed for stealing £1, was among these 27 suicides.[7]

To understand what shaped this recent British trend toward greater incarceration of women and its human consequences, in this chapter we examine the history of ideas about madness, mental illness, and mental health that have informed the perception, treatment, and control of prisoners, particularly women prisoners, in Britain. Feminist scholars have convincingly argued that women prisoners are subject to the language and ideas of psychiatry more than their male counterparts.[8-11] Furthermore, as this book aims to shift our understanding of women's incarceration away from their criminal identity toward their health needs, we wish to explore how an understanding of women's mental health care needs might be used to improve, rather than simply control, the lives of incarcerated women.

## THE BAD, MAD AND CRIMINALLY INSANE

The prison and asylum systems that took shape in nineteenth-century Britain were based on a firm distinction between badness and madness. Pathological conduct was understood and dealt with differently in each of these two regimes of confinement. Criminals were seen as responsible actors to be punished and corrected. In 1791, Bentham proposed a blueprint for modern prisons in his Panopticon, which would function as ". . . a mill to grind rogues honest and idle men [and presumably women too] industrious . . ."[12(p.26)] Though never built exactly as Bentham proposed, his Panopticon substantially influenced prison architecture and disciplinary regimes of nineteenth-century British prisons. Its radial architecture facilitated a hierarchal regime of unobtrusive surveillance, where senior guards observed their juniors who in turn observed the prisoners, to promote self-surveillance and self-discipline. Fifty-four prisons were built in this radial construction style during the 1840s alone, and these prisons routinely exerted regimes of work-based discipline and silent penitence on prisoners.

By contrast, lunatics, seen as lacking reason and responsibility, were given the peace and protection of asylum accompanied by moral treatment to enable them to recover their civility. Criminals were thought less eligible or deserving than lunatics, evident in the fact that far greater philanthropic zeal and optimism accompanied the founding of the British asylum system than did the development of prisons. However, the voting public did not support spending by local and central governments on either system – prisons or asylums – as this would have resulted in higher taxes. With few resources it was little wonder that both systems fell short of the goal of rehabilitation, and simply accumulated and warehoused persons with criminal histories and mental illness.

The differentiation between badness and madness, and the distinction between the two systems, was always problematic, with frequent attempts being made to place criminality under the domain of psychiatry. Darwinian degenerationist theory, which regarded the mad and criminal as genetically impaired beings, dominated late nineteenth-century psychiatry and criminology.[13,14] Both psychiatry and criminology studied pathological behaviors that they viewed as having the same root cause – genetics. Thus, were not the different forms of pathological behavior essentially the same? Surely knowledge from one discipline could be used to inform knowledge of the other. Such thinking informed the famous late nineteenth-century Italian criminologist Cesare Lambrosso as he conducted psychiatric studies of criminals.

Though psychiatric pathology could be recognized in criminality, the wholesale redefinition of criminals as mental patients was held in check by the invention of the intermediate category of criminal lunacy. People whose behavior was both clearly criminal and insane could be positioned in this category, allowing the distinction between the two forms of pathological behavior to continue. Following the 1800 Criminal Lunatic Act, criminal wings were added to lunatic asylums, before Broadmoor, the first criminal lunatic asylum, was opened in 1863. The criminal lunatic asylums, renamed special hospitals, became well established and eventually an embarrassingly anachronistic institution.

Gender always featured as a complex influence in the distinction between badness and madness. With considerable fluctuation in degree, men have outnumbered women as prisoners, whilst women, to a lesser extent, have outnumbered men in the psychiatric system. Yet, historically, women are not strangers to prison. When Britain stopped transporting prisoners to its colonies in 1867, the prison population swelled at home. The 1878 Prison Act reforms allowed some replacement of prison sentences with community supervision for less serious crimes and this facilitated the beginning of a sustained drop in Britain's prison population throughout the twentieth century to a low of 10 613, in 1936.[9] As women's crimes were generally less serious than those of men, the number of women sent to prison fell to 33 000 in 1913 and 11 000 in 1921.[15]

Furthermore, women have received separate and different treatment in the prisons of the modern age. John Howard, a prison reformer, substantially shaped many of the progressive developments of nineteenth-century prisons, through his book, *The State of Prisons in England and Wales*.[16] Howard argued for women to be kept away from the contaminating influence of lewd, rowdy men.

The Quaker prison reformist Elizabeth Fry also campaigned for special provisions to be made for women at Newgate prison in the 1840s, such as schools for children imprisoned with their mothers.[17]

Despite women's significant presence in prison, some have speculated that deviant behavior in men is more readily identified as criminal, whilst in women it is more readily recognized as mental disorder.[18] In a study comparing female and male violent offenders in Britain, Allen[19] concludes that legal decisions are constantly biased in favor of female offenders, particularly in relation to seriously violent crime. Allen argues that a sort of "chivalry" exists as psychiatric and legal professionals routinely make decisions that dissolve the guilt of violent women, transforming them into pitiful victims requiring leniency, whilst men, despite being ascribed mental pathologies, are sent to prison. Though such gender bias might work in the case of serious crime, it clearly did not work for the large number of women sent to prison at the turn of the twentieth century or for those increasingly being sentenced to prison today who, as in the case of Leanne Gidney, might only be guilty of petty crime. However, as Bartlett[20] points out, more psychiatric pathology is recognized and treated in the female prison population than in the male prison population. Furthermore, women in prison are also more likely to have been in contact with psychiatric services prior to conviction. Perhaps this simply confirms Chesler's[21] contention that femininity is culturally associated with madness; therefore, women more readily receive psychiatric diagnoses and treatment. As Busfield[22] subsequently argued, women's higher psychiatric morbidity may not be entirely the outcome of socially constructed diagnoses but could reflect their higher incidence of mental suffering, brought about by social disadvantage within a patriarchal society. To individualize women's mental health problems and identify them as psychiatric pathologies when they are really the result of their social disadvantage is misleading and depoliticizing.

## THE THERAPEUTIC PRISON

Gradual but sustained reforms to prisons from the late nineteenth century to the mid-twentieth century helped promote ideas and practices of the therapeutic, rather than the punitive, prison. Wardens, renamed prison officers in 1919, received their first training in 1935. Volunteer teachers began working in prisons during the 1920s and, thereafter, training and rehabilitation schemes gradually developed. The flogging of prisoners was eventually abolished in 1948.[23]

This therapeutic orientation toward prisoners enabled some degree of redefinition of criminal behavior as mental illness. Mid-twentieth-century changes in the psychiatric system itself gave rise to these changes in orientation. Psychiatric drugs, more widely used in society, became available in prisons. Although the press viewed this practice as a means of control rather than treatment, many prisoners were already receiving psychiatric drugs before admission and often actively demanded these drugs as a means of coping with the mental suffering of prison.[24] The greater use of psychiatric drugs was just one of many changes within the reorganization of the psychiatric system to have an effect within prisons. Asylums were being renamed mental hospitals and lunatics referred to as mental patients. In these more open institutions, new treatment regimes, known as social psychiatry, gave rise to the development of community care. The Mental Health Act 1959 reflected these major changes, and its main feature was to establish voluntary admission to and treatment in mental hospitals as the norm. The Act also established a new category of mental disorder – psychopathy – with which psychiatrists could legitimately treat individuals, even under compulsion. People, hitherto regarded as bad, rather irresponsible, yet not overtly mad, could now be regarded as having the mental disorder of psychopathy. If deemed treatable by psychiatrists, a psychopath could be detained and treated in a mental hospital. This treatability clause meant that psychiatrists controlled the entrance to and exit from mental hospitals for psychopaths, allowing psychiatrists to select prisoners they wished to treat. Those identified as treatable psychopaths tended to be placed in the special hospitals that now stood out as grim reminders of the bygone age of asylum confinement. With the development of forensic mental health care as a specialist practice, the special hospitals gradually reformed and gave rise to smaller secure units that partially replaced them. Some 3159 men and 442 women are now incarcerated as mental patients in this burgeoning forensic mental health care system of secure units and special hospitals.[25]

During these reforms, perhaps psychiatry's largest change was not the treatment of prisoners with psychiatric medications or the establishment of psychopathy as a mental disorder but rather its broadening mandate to treat normality itself through generalized intervention.[26] Just as social work moved beyond an exclusive attention to those in poverty, so too did psychiatry move beyond exclusively treating those with mental illness.

Everybody's mental health became the business of psychiatry, a philosophy increasingly endorsed within government mental health care policies and symptomatic of this high point of welfare liberalism. Britain's post Second World War welfare state emphasized principles of social democracy that encouraged the rethinking of women's role in society and social reform for disadvantaged and marginal groups, such as women prisoners.

These events led to women's prison reform in Britain during the late 1960s. With the nation's prison population at an extremely low level, women had become an anomalous rarity there. The thousand or so women prisoners were moved from prison wings, too small to be viable, into a few women's prisons. In London, Holloway became the main women's prison and the centre of this reform.[27] Given so few women, the task of turning the female prison service around did not seem insurmountable. Women prisoners became more marginal within the prison system and politically less visible as media stories and inquiries were preoccupied with men escaping. Therefore, the Holloway prison reform could occur without any public backlash. Within the prison service, reformers argued that the nineteenth-century radial prison was outmoded and unsuitable for the practice of progressive penology. Progressive penology meant doing away with roll calls, prisoner uniforms, hierarchical discipline, and high security in favor of psychotherapy and rehabilitation. The prison building, seen as the main obstacle, was replaced by a building that looked and functioned more like a hospital, which the reformers hoped it might eventually become. The central observation point of the radial prison was to be replaced by a green space and the straight-line prison wings replaced with undulating bands of small units. Psychoanalytical group therapy and individual casework were to replace psychiatric drugs and block treatment of the hierarchal disciplinary order. The proposed reform had widespread support from politicians of the day with only one critical voice of dissent from the abolitionist Anne Smith:

> . . . who argued quietly that, whilst the demolition of the old Holloway prison was to be commended, and the new Holloway's emphasis on rehabilitation was to be applauded, imprisoning women was so ill-advised that there should be no plans for a new establishment at all.[27(p.107)]

The Holloway project had limited success. Demolition and rebuilding were slow and imperfect as finances dwindled. When the new prison was finally finished 20 years later, prison staff went on strike, concerned about managing safety within the new regime. This long and difficult project failed to be the marvel reformers had hoped for, as by then they had moved on. As Rock[27] explains, the staff had lost memory, interest and understanding of the reform they had inherited.

Characteristics of the old Holloway, including high security, humiliating disciplinary practices (such as strip searches), poor medical care, and routine prescription of psychotropic drugs, now also characterized the new Holloway. Furthermore, the reformers' plan had depended on the women prisoner population continuing to decline. In fact, numbers increased slightly as the project proceeded and then rose sharply from the mid-1990s, ensuring that Holloway remained a prison rather than becoming a quasi-hospital alternative.

The failure of the Holloway reformist project must also be understood in the wider social context of a shift in Britain from welfare liberalism to advanced liberalism. A radical right wing government took power in 1979 and stridently dismantled and reorganized the welfare state, whilst encouraging economic freedom and individuality by deregulating markets and lowering taxes. Unemployment soared in the 1980s, though later leveled off and declined. Progressively Britain became a more divided society between those who benefited from the new free market enterprise society and those whom it marginalized. In this more unequal society crime rates increased, which in time led the government to enact tougher policies to control crime. Initially, the Conservative government, concerned to reduce the tax burden of the prison service, developed privatization policies and reduced the prison popu-lation. However, these policies eventually gave way to tougher talk in 1993, when the Home Secretary proclaimed that prison worked, arguing that it protected the public from wrongdoers and deterred many tempted to commit crime.[28] From that time, the prison population, particularly that of women, seriously increased.

## THE HEALTHY PRISON

Despite a change of government in 1997, no slow-down occurred in this upward trend. One of the most famous sound bites of the New Labour Prime Minister, Tony Blair, was "tough on crime, tough on the causes of crime,"[29] which in prac-tice involved a mixture of authoritarian law and order policies whilst appearing to be rather liberal. In contrast to the earlier Conservative Home Secretary, New Labour's Jack Straw declared "prison doesn't work, but we'll make it work."[28(p.229)] In practice this meant more imprisonment with longer sentences to punish wrongdoers and, on the other hand, policies aimed at improving prison-ers' health and well-being. Recent public health policy[30] focuses on the need for healthy prisons. One might well ask how the compulsory detention of anyone, causing them to lose their partner, children, home, job, and self-esteem, can do anything but harm a person's health. Although one could dismiss this phrase as an oxymoron, the Labour government should be unequivocally congratulated for its policy of transferring the responsibility for the health care of prisoners from the prison system to the health care trusts of the National Health Service (NHS).[30] The NHS is the publicly funded health care system of Britain. Trusts are statutory bodies responsible for delivering health care and health improve-ment to local areas. Though it might take time for implementation, there is now a clear policy that insists that prisoners have the same standard of health care as others within a health care trust catchment area. Already the policy has provided prisoners with health services from midwives and community nurses, who offer the same type and standard of health care to prisoners as is given to people in the community.

However, delivering the same type of mental health care in prison that is offered to people in the community may reveal the new policy's limitations. As in many other nations, recent mental health programs in British prisons have been informed by the "What Works" philosophy. This movement is an attempt to operate only programs that have an evidence base purportedly proven to reduce reoffending. These rehabilitative interventions claim to adhere to four key principles.

1  The Risk Principle: it is essential that reliable risk assessments of reoffending are undertaken because individuals at greater risk require more intensive programs.
2  The Need Principle: programs should focus upon only those qualities that are statistically associated with recidivism and relatively stable but still changeable. These predictors of future criminal conduct are associated with deficit or faulty thinking.
3  Responsivity: the delivery approach should match the learning styles of offenders. Cognitive behavioral programs are claimed to be effective.
4  Integrity: programs should be conducted in a structured way with strict adherence to the program manual.

In accordance with these principles, risk/needs assessments and highly structured, prepackaged treatment modules based on cognitive behavioral psychological methods, which encourage people to use reasoned thinking rather than emotions to motivate their actions, now dominate British prisons. With titles such as "Think First, Reasoning and Rehabilitation" and "Enhanced Thinking Skills," programs generally assume that criminal behavior is the consequence of faulty or deficient thinking and aim to inculcate new thinking skills or restructure cognitions.

Scholars have increasingly challenged the evidence base underlying these practices.[31] Feminists have argued that much research and evaluation carried out under the "What Works" rubric, relies heavily upon samples of young, white American males and does not transfer to women, other ethnic/racial groups, older populations, and members of other nations.[32] Furthermore "What Works" programs focus on the purported inadequacies of individuals while neglecting the broader social structure. An example of this process is evident in a Home Office report detailing a new strategy for women offenders:

> For this authoritarian government, promising to be tough on crime and its causes, there is no excuse for crime, whatever a person's background or experience. However, the characteristics of women prisoners suggest that experiences such as poverty, abuse and drug addiction lead some women to believe that their options are limited. Many offending behaviour programmes are designed to help offenders see that there are always positive choices open to them that do not involve crime. At the same time, across Government, we are tackling the aspects of social exclusion that make some women believe their options are limited.[3(p.7)]

The assumption of the "What Works" paradigm is that women have unlimited options and if they believe otherwise they simply have faulty thinking. From this perspective, social structural barriers are unchallenged. Furthermore, this logic uses women's adverse social circumstances, such as poverty and abuse, against them by claiming that such experiences lead them to distorted thinking and, consequently, to irresponsible choices including criminal behavior.

In response to these criticisms, and in recognition that women's pathways to crime and program needs are different than those of men, a number of feminists have recently recommended gender-specific programming.[32] This marks a shift from "What Works" to "What Works With Women." While the intention of gender-sensitive approaches is laudable and crucial to the establishment of a more humane penal regime, recent attempts to introduce gender-responsive programming have been problematic.

For example, Dialectical Behavior Therapy (DBT) was introduced as a less stigmatizing cognitive behavioral program designed to meet the needs of women diagnosed with Borderline Personality Disorder (BPD). Yet, as Warner[33] argues, the label of BPD is given to women who challenge gender role stereotypes, and BPD is a new name for an old problem – disorderly women.

Developed by the American psychologist Marcia Linehan as a treatment for BPD among her patients in the community, the main goals of DBT are to change rigid thinking and to instill emotional regulation. However, some feminist writers have argued that when introduced into the prison environment DBT may operate as a coercive and punitive management tool rather than as therapy. For example, distress tolerance is a DBT technique designed to help people deal with heightened emotions, such as fear, anger and frustration. However, within the prison system, it may be used as a means to silence protest against unfair or unjust practices.[31]

The example of DBT illustrates the dangers of co-optation when programs, however well intended, are introduced into the prison environment. The possibility for empowerment and rehabilitation is questionable under a regime characterized by unequal power relations, surveillance and extreme loss of control.

## SUMMARY AND CONCLUSION

The harmful effects of imprisonment are compounded by the fact that programs for female prisoners have tended to focus on women's psychology in a manner that reframes issues of unequal power relations, poverty, and violence as problems rooted in the individual. Perhaps we need to focus less on the mental pathology of women in prison to consider the shortcomings and irrationality of the policies of the various modes of liberalism that have attempted to address their psychiatric/criminogenic needs. Perhaps we need to reflect on the astute words of Friedrich Nietzsche: "Madness is rare in individuals – but in groups, political parties, nations, and ages it is the rule."[34(p.156)]

## REFERENCES

1 Downes D. The macho penal economy. Mass incarceration in the US: a European perspective. In: Giddens A, editor. *The Global Third Way Debate.* Cambridge: Polity Press; 2001. pp. 210–23.

2 Her Majesty's Prison Service. *Prison Population Bulletin December 22, 2006.* pp. 20. Available at: www.hmprisonservice.gov.uk/resourcecentre/publicationsdocuments/index.asp?startrow=101&cat=85&id=166,154,1,166,0,0, (accessed May, 2009).

3 Home Office. *Statistics on Women and the Criminal Justice System 2001.* London: Home Office; 2002.

4 Home Office. *Prison Statistics England and Wales 2001.* London: The Stationery Office; 2003.

5 Home Office. *Female Prisoners 2006.* Available at: www.hmprisonservice.gov.uk/adviceandsupport/prison_life/femaleprisoners (accessed November 2, 2008).

6 www.womeninprison.org.uk

7 Sim J. At the centre of the new professional gaze: women, medicine and confinement. In: Chan W, Chunn DE, Menzies R, editors. *Women, Madness and the Law: a feminist reader.* London: Routledge Cavendish; 2005. pp. 211–25.

8 Carlen P. Law, psychiatry and women's imprisonment: a sociological view. *Br J Psychiatry.* 1985; **146**: 618–21.

9 Sim J. *Medical Power in Prisons: the prison medical service in England 1774–1989.* Milton Keynes: Open University Press; 1990.

10 Worrall A. *Offending Women: female lawbreakers and the criminal justice system.* London: Routledge; 1990.

11 Chan W, Chunn DE, Menzies R. *Women, Madness and the Law: a feminist reader.* London: Routledge Cavendish; 2005.

12 Scull A. *Decarceration: community treatment and the deviant – a radical view.* 2nd ed. Cambridge: Polity Press; 1984.

13 Sampson C. Madness and psychiatry. In: Turner B, editor. *Medical Power and Social Knowledge.* 2nd ed. London: Sage Publications; 1995. pp. 55–83.

14 Porter R. *Madness: a brief history.* Oxford: Oxford University Press; 2002.

15 Smith A. *Women in Prison: a study in penal methods.* London: Stevens; 1962.

16 Howard J. *The State of Prisons in England and Wales.* London: Cadell & Conant; 1784.

17 Carlen P, Worrall A. *Analysing Women's Imprisonment.* Devon: Willan Publishing; 2004.

18 Smart C. *Women, Crime and Criminology: a feminist critique.* London: Routledge and Kegan Paul; 1976.

19 Allen H. *Justice Unbalanced: gender, psychiatry and judicial decisions.* Milton Keynes: Open University Press; 1987.

20 Bartlett A. *Expert Paper: social division and difference: women.* Liverpool: NHS National Programme on Forensic Mental Health Research and Development; 2002.

21 Chesler P. *Women and Madness.* New York, NY: Doubleday; 1972.

22 Busfield J. *Men, Women and Madness: understanding gender and mental disorder*. London: Macmillan; 1996.

23 The Howard League for Penal Reform. *A Short History of Prison*. 2008. Available at: www.howardleague.org/index.php?id=31 (accessed February 17, 2009).

24 Carlen P. Psychiatry in prison: promises, premises, practices and politics. In: Miller P, Rose N, editors. *The Power of Psychiatry*. Cambridge: Polity Press; 1986. pp. 241–66.

25 Ministry of Justice. *Statistics of Mentally Disordered Offenders 2006*. 7 December 2007: Ministry of Justice Statistical Bulletin. Available at: http://noms.justice.gov.uk/news-publications-events/publications/newsletters/mdobulletin?view=Binary (accessed May 25, 2009).

26 Castel R. From dangerousness to risk. In: Burchell G, Gordon C, Miller P, editors. *The Foucault Effect: studies in governmentality*. London: Harvester Wheatsheaf; 1991. pp 281–98.

27 Rock P. *Reconstructing a Women's Prison: the Holloway redevelopment project 1968–88*. Oxford: Clarendon Press; 1996.

28 Carlen P. New discourses of justification and reform for women's imprisonment in England. In: Carlen P, editor. *Women and Punishment: the struggle for justice*. Devon: Willan Publishing; 2002. pp. 220–36.

29 Blair T. Speech at the Labour Party Conference, Brighton. 1992.

30 Department of Health. *Health Promoting Prisons: a shared approach*. London: Department of Health; 2002.

31 Kendall K, Pollack S. Cognitive behaviouralism in women's prisons: a critical analysis of therapeutic assumptions and practices. In: Bloom B, editor. *Gendered Justice: addressing female offenders*. Durham, NC: Carolina Academic Press; 2003. pp. 69–96.

32 Bloom B, Owen B, Covington S, *et al. Gender-Responsive Strategies: research, practice, and guiding principles for women offenders*. Washington, DC: National Institute of Corrections; 2003. Available at: www.nicic.org/pubs/2003/018017.pdf (accessed February 17, 2009).

33 Warner S. Visibly special? Women, child sexual abuse and special hospitals. In: Hemingway C, editor. *Special Women? The Experience of Women in the Special Hospital System*. Aldershot: Avebury; 1996. pp. 59–72.

34 Nietzsche F. *Beyond Good and Evil*. London: Penguin; 2003.

# CHAPTER 6

# The Importance of Gender in US Prisons

Nancy Stoller

This chapter explores the ways that gender is managed through prison policies and practices. I compare and contrast the treatment of women and men, through an approach that pays specific attention to racism and ethnicity, with an emphasis on African-American, Latino/a, Native American and white prisoners in the US.

The primary focus is on institutional management and control as affected by race, gender, and class in the following areas: prisoners' backgrounds, classification on arrival and living conditions, access to services (including health care), childbirth and parenting, gender and sexual management, violence, release, and parole. This contextualization of women's experiences in prison is important for two main reasons: first, so that readers will not homogenize "the woman prisoner," ignoring differences among women that are institutionally consequential; and secondly, so they will not generalize from women's experiences of prison and prison health to the lives of men in prison or imagine that women's prison experiences can be understood through a lens that focuses primarily on men.

## PRISONERS' BACKGROUNDS

The majority of all prisoners are poor people of color. Institutionalized racism spans a process of criminalization that includes lack of educational, financial and social opportunities; racial profiling; police brutality; inequities in sentencing; racism inside US prisons; disparities in parole policies; and discrimination faced by people with felony records.[1] The racialized aspect of the criminal justice system is pronounced for both women and men. In 2006 African-American women were incarcerated at a rate that is 3.1 times that of white women, and African-American men at a rate of 6.2 that of white men.[2]

Disproportionate confinement of people of color should be understood within the US national context of institutionalized racism. A "systems" approach to examining the criminal justice system views prisons and jails as institutions of social control. Such an approach also views the criminal justice system as a contributor to institutional racism. The criminal justice system dissolves families and directly affects the larger communities of the families. The multi-generational impact of prison on children and parents of prisoners further devastates poor people and communities of color.[3] Women prisoners are at the nexus of this impact and therefore should be a key focus in the interventions that can reduce the effects of prisons/incarceration on communities. Improving the health and reducing the number of women incarcerated can have enorm-ous positive impacts on nuclear and extended families because the majority of incarcerated women have children under 18.

In their 2005 study of the impact of the contemporary drug prosecutions on women, the ACLU found that:

> . . . even when they have minimal or no involvement whatsoever in the drug trade, women are increasingly caught in the ever widening net cast by current drug laws through provisions such as conspiracy, accomplice liability and con-structive possession, that expand criminal liability to reach partners, relatives, and bystanders. Sentencing laws fail to consider the many reasons – including domestic violence, economic dependence, or dependent immigration status – that may compel women to remain silent or not to report a partner or family member's drug activity to authorities. Moreover, existing sentencing policies, particularly mandatory minimum laws, often subject women to the same, or in some cases, harsher sentences than the principals in the drug trade who are ostensibly the target of those policies.[4(p.4)]

The rate of imprisonment for women varies from state to state as well as by region because of a number of reasons including use of alternatives to incarcera-tion, sentencing guidelines, judicial discretion regarding family responsibilities, and parole board policies. For example, approximately 129 of every 100 000 women in Oklahoma are serving state prison sentences while Massachusetts imprisons only 11 women for every 100 000 female state residents. In California, the incarceration rate is 61 per 100 000 women residents. Between 1977 and 2004 the number of women in California state prisons grew by 1522%, and even though the growth in numbers has slowed somewhat since 1999, it is still in an upward trajectory.[5]

In their review of incarceration patterns for women over the past 30 years, the Institute on Women and Criminal Justice of the Women's Prison Association[5] found four distinct themes to describe the etiology of women's criminal behaviors and their personal and social problems.

> First, most women in the criminal justice system come from neighborhoods that are entrenched in poverty and largely lacking in viable systems of social support. Second, alarmingly large numbers of these women have experienced very serious physical and/or sexual abuse, often commencing when they were young children. Third, as adults, most of these women are plagued with high levels of physical and mental health problems as well as substance abuse issues. Often these problems are combined and compounded. Fourth, the great majority of the women who have suffered from these deprivations, histories of trauma and abuse, and health deficits are mothers – and they are far more likely than men in the criminal justice system to be the sole support and caregivers for their children.[5(pp.21,22), see also 6–9]

The Women's Prison Association takes an optimistic view regarding future growth of prison populations, citing national trends since 2000:

> While some states, as well as the federal criminal justice system, still remain on the same 'get tough' course, a handful of states have turned the corner and begun to significantly downsize their prison systems.[5(p.27)]

Indeed, efforts in a few states to reduce reliance on incarceration suggest that just as the get-tough excesses of the 1980s and 1990s have had great impact on women, strategies that reverse some of this legislation should bring specific relief for women. For example, in 2000 California voters approved a drug diversion program (Proposition 36) that has kept tens of thousands of people arrested for possession of drugs out of prison.[10] The number of women sentenced to prison dropped by 10% in the first year, and correctional managers named Proposition 36 as the largest factor driving the decline.[11] Early in 2003 the Department of Corrections was able to close the Northern California Women's Facility at Stockton, and the state saved $500 million by delaying construction of new prisons during 2003–4.[10] In May 2007, however, California Governor Arnold Schwarzenegger signed legislation to expand the state prison system by 40 000 new prison beds and 13 000 new county jail beds, of which an unknown number will be for women. The new women's units are expected to be located closer to major population centers than the state's larger prisons. Some new units may provide special accommodations to allow women to have their children with them. Although the rate of female incarceration may drop with national and state changes in sentencing and diversion programs, a number of researchers predict that the incarceration rate for women in the US will be stable at 5–15% of the total number of prisoners.[2,12]

## CLASSIFICATION ON ARRIVAL AND LIVING CONDITIONS

Arrival in prison for both men and women begins with classification. As Foucault noted in his classic study of the emergence of prisons in Western societies, prisons operate by labeling, categorizing, processing, and socializing in order to produce a class of people who are known as prisoners.[13] Once the new arrival has become a prisoner, this label and social identity remains throughout one's life, along with its stigmatizing and legal consequences.

Basic classification includes the level of security required for confinement: minimum, medium, high security; super max; fire camp, etc. Because there are smaller numbers of women prisoners, there are fewer women's institutions spread out over larger distances. Therefore, security classification can be quite different. Men who are low security risks have a much greater chance of being housed in low or minimum security institutions; women are more frequently housed in settings designated as medium and maximum level. Consequences of this disparity range from ease of visiting by family, access to appropriate programs, and daily living conditions. When we remember that most women are serving sentences for non-violent offenses, we can see that they are also typically in more restrictive environments than men.[14,15]

Unlike male prisoners, women are not typically housed by ethnic or racial category.[16] Primary consideration is given to security level. Racism still operates in the culture via guards' treatment of women: in many institutions racist language is tolerated, Spanish and other non-English speakers have limited ability to find someone in authority who understands them, and privileges are more accessible to white women.[17] The best jobs are given to the best educated, and certain manual work (e.g. unit cleaning, kitchen or laundry) may be assigned to African-Americans and Latinas who often experience discrimination. This has many consequences, including reinforcement of economic disparities, since even at the low pay scale of prison work some jobs pay nothing while others range on a scale that rewards the most elite of the population.[18]

## ACCESS TO SERVICES

Prison services are designed for the majority of prisoners, who are men. Consequently, many services that women need are provided as afterthoughts. For example, obstetrical and gynecological services may be limited or hard to access. Arrangements for mother-infant visits are a low priority. While women are predominantly in prison for drug-related matters and most have histories of substance abuse, alcoholism, violence, rape, and homelessness, programs to address these needs are rare. In addition, even when rehabilitative or training programs are provided, their approach may be more appropriate for men.[19]

## CHILDBIRTH AND PARENTING

The majority of women prisoners are mothers to children under 18. Incarceration separates mothers from their families, often leaving them despondent over the loss of their children.[20]

Legal Services for Prisoners with Children (LSPC), an advocacy organization in California, summarizes the threat to parenting when women are incarcerated:

> The incarceration of women uniquely impacts families and communities because women are often the primary caregivers of children. Additionally, because the prison industrial complex disproportionately impacts people of color, Black, Latino and Native children are at a greater risk for losing a parent to incarceration. When a man goes to prison, wives, sisters, mothers, grandmothers, and aunts often work to keep the family together. When a woman goes to prison – and there is no one able to care for her child – she runs the risk of losing her parental rights, meaning she no longer has any legal rights regarding her child. Too often, thousands of children end up as wards of the state and are shuffled throughout the foster care system. More still are adopted out, never to see their incarcerated parent again.[21]

## THE MANAGEMENT OF GENDER PRESENTATION AND SEXUALITY

It is generally agreed that transgender male-to-female (MTF) women in male prisons are at high risk.[22] In a 2006 California study, Jenness, *et al.*[23] found that 59% of the state's transgender MTF prisoners reported being sexually assaulted, compared with 4% of the general prison population. Other non-heterosexual inmates and black inmates were considerably more vulnerable to sexual assault as well. In a striking difference concerning medical responsiveness, prisoners reported that in the majority of assaults on members of the general prison population, guards were aware of the attack and medical care was provided when needed, but when the victim was transgendered, the guards were often unaware and medical care, even when needed, was not provided. A major reason for this appears to lie in a lack of reporting by either the transgender victims or other witnesses. The American Public Health Association has proposed methods of notification about sexual assault, as well as assault prevention strategies, that may reduce the risk of further violence for victims and witnesses.[24]

Jenness' study[23] did not include transgender female-to-male (FTM) men in prison. In fact the invisibility of this population to researchers may be partly understood by the reverse meanings of transgender in the sexist world of prisons. MTF transgender identity is understood as a move toward passivity, receptivity, weakness, and stigmatizing femininity within an environment that demands masculinity. FTM is the opposite: the identification with the more valued masculine persona. Although FTM persons and butch lesbians in women's prisons may be harassed by guards, they may also occupy higher status roles within the community of women prisoners.[16,25]

Prison rules often include detailed requirements for dress, make-up, and hairstyle according to gender. Historically, the US has had two types of women's prisons: reformatories, primarily for white women who were seen as having fallen off the path to respectability; and custodial prisons that were filled with women of color who were stereotyped by administrators and politicians as dangerous.[26] Since the late twentieth-century rise of more punitive prisons and a concomitant growth in the proportion of African-American, Latina/o, and Native prisoners, the majority of US facilities are of the custodial type. In the reformatory, skirts might have been required and masculine style forbidden; in the punitive custodial setting, women may be purposely dressed in drab colors, jeans, tees, and sweatshirts or in prison uniforms in garish colors. They are often forbidden jewelry and long or dyed hair. While women still adjust their assigned appearances for individuality and the specific type of gender presentation or sexual message they may wish to convey, they can also be disciplined for these adaptations. For men, there are similar bans on "looking like women." Men may also be required to shave (unless they can present a doctor's prescription indicating how this might harm their skin), forbidden to wear a moustache, and punished for wearing scarves or other feminine attire. Men who dress in feminine styles are often blamed if they are the victims of sexual assault.[27]

Consensual sexual behavior between prisoners is banned in both men's and women's prisons. Many commentators have argued that women's sex in prison is the outcome of intimacy and affection, while sex between incarcerated men is the result of exploitation.[25,28] However, other studies and prisoners' own writings indicate that love can exist anywhere and that women are just as capable of exploitative relationships in prison as are men.[16,27]

Prisoners can be punished for hugging or touching either by authorities or by other prisoners. In the case of men, the prisoner-to-prisoner punishment (i.e. violence) rarely results in any discipline and may be followed by more violence from other prisoners and/or guard harassment.

Prison visiting rooms are replete with warnings and enforcement preventing touching, kissing, hugging, and anything that approaches sex. In California prisons, for example, the only kisses allowed are one at the start and one at the end of the visit and even these must be chaste. Throughout the US, private conjugal visits are only allowed in six states, but not in federal prisons. California announced in June 2008 that it would also allow gay or lesbian couples overnight visiting rights.[29]

## VIOLENCE

Violence in women's prisons is less evident or documented than in men's prisons. Guard violence is less deadly with far fewer shootings. However, women prisoners do fight, harass, and exploit each other's weaknesses. Additionally, they may be pressed into sexual relationships with guards against their will.

In 2003, the Federal Prison Rape Elimination Act[30] was signed into law. However, minimal change followed, with the primary funding going to research. A few programs have been initiated on the state level. For example, the state of Ohio has begun a 10-point program with the goal of reducing prison rape and sexual assault to zero. The major aspects of the program are: staff training; inmate education; sanctions; victim support persons; investigation procedures; data collection; audits; and process improvement teams to address fear of reporting. Some states have passed similar laws.

## RELEASE AND STAYING OUT

People who have been incarcerated are usually desperately poor on release. They encounter all the barriers that low and no income people face plus the additional stigma of having been in prison. It is extremely difficult for ex-prisoners, especially Latina/os and African-Americans, to find employment and housing and obtain public assistance. Even minimum and below-living wage jobs may be out of their reach. At the same time, current parole and policing policies make it much harder for them to stay on the right side of the law than it is for those without a criminal record. In effect, the system punishes people for life instead of for the time period of their incarceration.

One approach to improve the chances of reintegration that is often espoused is the use of reentry programs. Research suggests that programs located in communities, lasting more than six months, focusing on people with a high risk of parole failure, providing vocational services, and using positive reinforcement could help more individuals stay out of prison. Successful programs with these components could reduce recidivism rates by 30%.[31]

Many existing public services, civil rights, and opportunities are not accessible to former prisoners due to discrimination. Both explicit and indirect discrimination prevents many from accessing services or participating fully in society.[3] Some examples of these discriminatory policies are: state bans that prohibit persons with felony convictions from voting; US federal policy of a lifetime denial of access to welfare for persons convicted of drug crimes, especially damaging to women; lack of access to housing, medical coverage, employment assistance, drug treatment and family reunification services; employment discrimination by private businesses and public agencies.[32,33]

## CONCLUSION

This chapter has argued that US prisons play a major role in the reinforcement of racism and sexism. Incarceration and its consequences are damaging to all prisoners, even though the methods and brutality may vary. When prisoners become ill or suffer unintended or intentional trauma, they are already in a hostile environment where their identities, former lives, families, affectional ties, and self-agency are at risk.

Consequently, when designing policies, programs, and trainings to improve health care for women in jails and prisons, it is important to remember that racism and sexism are part of the context, and present barriers to jail and prison health.[24] Without understanding how prisons handle gender and race, health service changes and clinical interventions may have limited impact.

## REFERENCES

1 Legal Services for Prisoners with Children. *All of Us or None.* 2008. Available at: www. allofusornone.org (accessed June 19, 2009).

2 Sabol WJ, Minton TD, Harrison PM. *Prison and Jail Inmates at Midyear 2006.* Washington, DC: Bureau of Justice Statistics; 2007. Available at: www.ojp.usdoj.gov/bjs/pub/pdf/pjim06.pdf (accessed December 16, 2008).

3 Mauer M, Chesney-Lind M, editors. *Invisible Punishment: the collateral consequences of mass imprisonment.* New York, NY: New Press; 2002.

4 Lapidus L, Luthra N, Verma A, *et al. Caught in the Net: the impact of drug policies on women and families.* 2005. Available at: www.aclu.org/drugpolicy/gen/23513pub20050315. html (accessed December 16, 2008).

5 Frost NA, Green J, Pranis K. Institute on Women and Criminal Justice. *The Punitiveness Report: Hard Hit: the growth in the imprisonment of women, 1977–2004.* 2006. Available at: www.wpaonline.org/institute/hardhit/index.htm (accessed December 16, 2008).

6 Raeder MS. The forgotten offenders: the effect of sentencing guidelines and mandatory minimums on women and their children. *Federal Sentencing Reporter.* 1995; 8: 157–62.

7 Browne A, Miller B, Maguin E. Prevalence and severity of lifetime physical and sexual victimization among incarcerated women. *Int J Law Psychiatry.* 1999; 22(3–4): 301–22.

8 Richie B. *Compelled to Crime: the gender entrapment of battered black women.* New York, NY: Routledge; 1996.

9 Chesney-Lind M. *The Female Offender: girls, women and crime.* 2nd ed. Thousand Oaks, CA: Sage Publications; 2004.

10 Drug Policy Alliance. *Prop. 36 Has Cut Prison Costs, Populations – Fact Sheet.* 2004. Available at: www.prop36.org/prop36_fact_sheet.html (accessed December 16, 2008).

11 Mark M. Changing population behind bars: major drop in women in state prisons: drug-rehab law called reason for 10% decline in past year. *San Francisco Chronicle.*

April 21, 2002. Available at: www.sfgate.com/cgi-bin/article.cgi?f=/c/a/2002/04/21/MN233500.DTL&type=printable (accessed December 16, 2008).

12 Walmsley R. *World Female Imprisonment List*. London: International Centre for Prison Studies; 2006. Available at: www.unodc.org/pdf/india/womens_corner/women_prison_list_2006.pdf (accessed December 16, 2008).

13 Foucault M. *Discipline and Punish: the birth of the prison*. New York, NY: Random House; 1977.

14 Human Rights Watch. *All Too Familiar: sexual abuse of women in US state prisons*. 1996. Available at: www.hrw.org/en/news/1996/12/06/sexual-abuse-women-us-state-prisons (accessed May 25, 2009).

15 Hoeflinger MM. All too familiar: sexual abuse of women in US state prisons, and nowhere to hide: retaliation against women in Michigan State Prisons. *Human Rights Quarterly*. 1999: **21**(1): 254–9.

16 Díaz-Cotto J. *Chicana Lives and Criminal Justice: voices from El Barrio*. Austin, TX: University of Texas Press; 2006.

17 Ross L. *Inventing the Savage: the social construction of Native American criminality*. Austin, TX: University of Texas Press; 1998.

18 California Coalition for Women Prisoners. *Critical Statistics*. 2008. Available at: www.womenprisoners.org/resources/critical_statistics.html (accessed December 16, 2008).

19 Beck JA. Recovering selves: women and the government of conduct in a therapeutic community. *Women & Therapy, A Feminist Quarterly*. 2006; **29**(3/4): 239–59.

20 Legal Services for Prisoners with Children. *Women Prisoners: facts and figures at a glance*. 2008. Available at: www.prisonerswithchildren.org/pubs/womgen.pdf (accessed May 25, 2009).

21 Legal Services for Prisoners with Children. *Overview*. 2008. Available at: www.prisonerswithchildren.org/issues/pwcover.htm (accessed December 16, 2008).

22 Peek C. Breaking out of the prison hierarchy: transgender prisoners, rape, and the Eighth Amendment. *Santa Clara Law Rev*. 2004; **44**: 1211–48.

23 Jenness V, Maxson CL, Matsuda KN, *et al*. *Violence in California Correctional Facilities: an empirical examination of sexual assault* [presentation]. 2007. Available at: www.nicic.org/Library/022407 (accessed December 16, 2008).

24 American Public Health Association. *Standards for Health Care in Jails and Prisons*. Washington, DC: American Public Health Association; 2003.

25 Faith K. *Unruly Women: the politics of confinement and resistance*. Vancouver, BC: Press Gang Publishers; 1993.

26 Freedman E. *Their Sisters' Keepers: women's prison reform in America, 1830–1930*. Ann Arbor, MI: University of Michigan Press; 1981.

27 Sabo D, Kupers TA, London W. *Prison Masculinities*. Philadelphia, PA: Temple University Press; 2001.

28 Ward D, Kassebaum G. *Women's Prison: sex and social structure*. Chicago, IL: Aldine Publishing; 1965.

29 Associated Press. *Calif. Gay, Lesbian Inmates Get Conjugal Visits*. Available at: www.msnbc.msn.com/id/18994457 (accessed December 16, 2008).

30 108th Congress. *Prison Rape Elimination Act of 2003. Public Law 108-79*. September 4, 2003. Available at: www.justdetention.org/pdf/PREA.pdf (accessed December 16, 2008).

31 Petersilia J. *Understanding California Corrections*. Berkeley, CA: California Policy Research Center, University of California; 2006. Available at: http://ucicorrections.seweb.uci.edu/pdf/UnderstandingCorrectionsPetersilia20061.pdf (accessed December 16, 2008).

32 The Sentencing Project. *Felony Disenfranchisement*. Available at: www.sentencingproject.org/IssueAreaHome.aspx?IssueID=4 (accessed December 16, 2008).

33 Allard P. *Life Sentences: denying welfare benefits to women convicted of drug offenses*. The Sentencing Project; 2002. Available at: www.sentencingproject.org/pdfs/9088.pdf (accessed December 16, 2008).

# CHAPTER 7

# Prisons Are Sickening: What Do We Do About It?

## Karlene Faith

Since the advent of criminology in the late nineteenth century, the rationales for building prisons have been to keep the public safe, deter prisoners from repeating offenses, deter others from breaking the law, and rehabilitate offenders as well as punish them, so as to induce law-abiding social values and behaviors. With the exception of punishment, prisons fail to achieve these objectives.[1,2]

Modern prisons were instituted over the course of the nineteenth century in the British Commonwealth nations and in the US as a substitute for the death penalty for all but heinous crimes.[1] Women in Canada were confined to a section of the men's federal penitentiary in Kingston, Ontario, in cold, dank, insect-ridden, foul-smelling cells 8½ feet x 30 inches. They were assaulted by guards, flogged for cursing, and punished for whatever else displeased their keepers. Throughout North America, beginning late in the century and accelerating in the 1950s, separate prisons were constructed for the relatively few women prisoners.[1]

In the twentieth century, prisoners were used by psychologists and psychiatrists as objects to be tested, measured, categorized, analyzed, labeled and treated with often harmful therapies. Pharmaceutical corporations tested out new drugs on prisoners, and by 1975 over half the women in many US prisons were inappropriately medicated.[3]

In the first decade of the twenty-first century, a global punishment industry has grown steadily, primarily warehousing those who lack the resources to defend themselves in court.[4,5] This industry includes multinational corporations that provide construction, security apparatus and the hundreds of goods, supplies and services required by total institutions. Often prisons are staffed by large unionized operations employing millions of people. Privatized prisons accrue profits with prisoner labor. In state-operated prisons, private contractors provide food, medical care, and all manner of services for a profit.

The first section of this chapter identifies how imprisonment damages women's physical, emotional, and mental health. Due to space limitations, I have included just a few brief quotes from women imprisoned in Canada and the US; these are drawn from my extensive research in women's prisons between 1972 and 2007. The second section discusses the ideals of restorative and transformational justice, and the abolition of imprisonment for people who pose no danger.

## THE EFFECTS OF PRISON ON WOMEN'S HEALTH

Incarceration is a health issue, routinely resulting in physical, mental, and emotional damage. Imprisoned women suffer overt and insidious harms that cannot be averted under conditions of forced confinement. "[M]ass incarceration is increasingly recognized as a public health issue . . . .. Jail and prison medical care is far below community standards of care and compromises the health and safety of prisoners and the community to which they will return."[6] The actual health conditions in most women's prisons fail to meet community standards and those outlined in the United Nations International Human Rights Standards for prisons. These include the order that medical officers regularly inspect prisons as to the quality of "food, water, hygiene, cleanliness, sanitation, heating, lighting, ventilation, clothing, bedding and opportunities for exercise . . . The primary responsibility of healthcare personnel is to protect the health of all prisoners."[7(pp.4–6)]

Following are examples of practices that are, or recently have been, routine in women's prisons in the US and Canada, and that negatively affect a woman's body as well as her emotional and mental health.

Inappropriate use of medications:

> They shoot you full of penicillin. They figure everyone has VD anyway so why bother with a test or pap smear, just shoot us full of penicillin.

Lack of adequate nutrition:

> Eggs? We won't have to worry about cholesterol. Two eggs a week. Fruit? Four pieces a week and a paucity of fresh vegetables. Milk? A little powdered milk poured out of a pitcher by an attendant on half a bowl of cereal for breakfast, and a cup (not a glass) of powdered milk for supper. This is a private food service and the company has to make a profit out of the prisoners.

Lack of access to proper hygiene supplies and living in dirty conditions:

> We have to buy what we need at the canteen, like tampons, toothpaste, shampoo, deodorant, all that stuff, but I don't have enough money so I go without things I need.
>
> They gave me a blanket but I got crabs from it. I was afraid to mention it because they would put me in the hole.

Exposure to infectious disease:

> I was infected when I came in and for seven weeks I walked around with it and they wouldn't do anything for me. Finally they diagnosed it and put me in isolation, but only after I'd been leaving the infection behind me everywhere for seven weeks.

The following are examples of common prison experiences that negatively affect women's mental health.

Concerns and fears for one's children:

> They put my daughter in a foster home as soon as I was arrested. My mother and husband came to get her but the welfare woman said my mother was "unfit." So they took my daughter to a foster home and said I couldn't have her and my family couldn't have her. I wouldn't sign the papers. Now my daughter is a ward of the court and I can't do anything about it. I can't pay a good lawyer. They've had her for a year. I can't concentrate. Once you pass through these gates there's nothing you can do about anything.

Working all day for an inadequate wage:

> We get $2.50 a day [*Can$, 2005*] for fulltime work. It costs 90 cents to make one phone call. All the items in the canteen cost more than they would outside and they are of the cheapest, poorest quality available. The prison won't allow anything to be brought in for the prisoners, anything at all. Everything the women need or want has to be bought from the canteen or done without. Isn't this a lovely setup for the private canteen company? – a captive group of women who are forced to buy the crappiest brands of everything for inflated prices.

Consequences of isolation and sensory deprivation:

> I was in a 5' × 8' isolation cell for a year, couldn't see if it was raining or snowing or what. Once a day I was allowed to walk in the corridor for ten minutes. You

go to the toilet in the same cell where you eat. I tried to commit suicide.

Not all women emotionally survive the prison experience, but some are resilient and manage it entirely alone, following the advice to "Do your own time." Some develop a supportive circle of friends and intimate relationships. A few women find a supportive member of the staff in whom they can confide. But others cut themselves off from others, or commit self-harm, or attempt and sometimes succeed at suicide.[8]

Emotions manifest what we call the spirit, soul or heart of a person, and prisons test a woman's spiritual fortitude in myriad ways.[2]

The pain of separation from children and worry for their welfare:

My baby has been separated from the older kids and I'm doing hard time around that. The foster parents won't bring her to see me because they say it would upset her. But the truth is she's upset because she can't see me or her older sisters. She's starting to stutter.

Difficulty sustaining communication with family and friends:

Visits, mail, phone calls are all censored and can be terminated any time. We never know how many years we will be here. Loneliness eats at your gut and you begin to vanish.

The stigma of being a criminal, a convict, an unworthy person, an outcast:

Numbered, stripped, searched, teeth counted, sprayed for bugs, I wanted to die. I was ill. I thought I would die.

Extreme, traumatic abuses against prisoners include routine internal body searches, which women experience as rape, sexual assault by guards, and stripping and chaining women in isolation. These and many other routine or circumstantial atrocities have been confirmed in North America by various court decisions, commissions, public hearings and inquiries.[8-12] The mistake is to think that prisons can be reformed. Imprisonment and healing are antithetical in part because prison relations are fundamentally adversarial. Power imbalances and abuses, arbitrary discipline, claustrophobia and paranoia all mitigate against the ideal of humanitarian reform. Prison confinement produces fear, tension, depression, anger, and/or a desire for revenge and brings out the worst in many, including prisoners, guards, and health care professionals. It is a conflicted environment by definition, inherently unhealthy.[1,2,13-17]

## FUTILITY OF REFORM: RESTORATIVE AND TRANSFORMATIVE JUSTICE

What, then, is to be done? Most crimes by women are non-violent drug-related offenses. To start, we need to transfer responsibility for drug policy to regulatory agencies and public health services.[18] An example of a pioneering step toward decriminalizing drug use is the highly successful Vancouver safe injection site and needle exchange program, cutting incidents of overdose and disease transmission, and encouraging recovery.[19]

Restorative justice aims to restore harmony by engaging the community in responding to the needs of victims and assuring that those who cause harm are held accountable while, at the same time, supporting their reintegration into the community. The victim is given restitution and care, the person who caused harm benefits from taking responsibility, and the community is strengthened in this process. In resolving the problem or conflict, cooperative community values are reinforced. A community may be a neighborhood, or people connected by heritage, religious beliefs, ethnicity, occupation, friendship or shared interests, and who, through those connections, form a community of care.

Formally instituted restorative justice programs within the criminal justice system are sometimes called "Alternative Dispute Resolution." Grassroots methods include different forms of mediation, community panels and healing circles in the traditions of Quakers, Mennonites and Aboriginals. In the 1980s, the Maori in New Zealand returned to the tradition of community and family group conferencing as the means of solving problems with youth, and the criminal justice system acknowledged their validity. The practice spread to Australia, was exported to Labrador and Newfoundland, and then spread across Canada. A fundamental distinction between court trials and restorative justice is that in a circle everyone's needs are recognized and everyone is heard. This is the appeal of restorative justice for those who take responsibility for the offense, victims who don't want to be invisible, and communities that value human relations. At any given restorative justice meeting, fewer than 20 people are likely to be directly involved in helping to find a resolution, but over time a majority of a community's members will have this experience, to settle their own conflicts, to serve as a support person for others involved, or to represent the community.[20]

Transformative justice is a critically analytical and activist variation on restorative justice, focusing on the ways that class, gender, ethnic and racial discriminations produce a fundamentally unjust social structure. The goal is to transform the political economy and hierarchical power structures to create a more equitable society, and to invest in health care, education, childcare, substance abuse treatment programs, job training, and social services rather than punishment. This requires a shift in the values that guide public policy and budget priorities. Restorative justice decreases the numbers of people locked up, and transformative justice promotes substantive change in the social structure.[20]

In Canadian communities with strong restorative justice programs, the police cooperate with, and sometimes make referrals to, local groups to resolve a problem instead of putting individuals in jail. The Royal Canadian Mounted Police have developed their own version of conferencing with all those with a stake in the outcome of a case, referred to as "community justice forums." The police involved in these programs present themselves as peacemakers and facilitators of social justice, rather than as gatekeepers for the prison system. Similarly, both the Canadian Department of Justice and the Law Commission advocate participatory justice to ensure that those most affected by a crime have an active voice in the resolution. Likewise, in 2002, the United Nations issued a declaration of basic principles on the use of restorative justice, urging all member states to implement programs.[7,20] Dozens of countries obliged.

Despite lack of funding, restorative approaches are evolving in the policy, academic and activist sectors simultaneous with, and as a response to, the steady global expansion of the prison industry. Prisons erode the communities from which most prisoners are drawn and to which they will return (*see* Chapter 2, Olesen). Restorative justice helps to rebuild communities and personal relations, and attend to those who have been victimized – which includes most prisoners. For example, a significant majority of women in prisons across North America have been victims of sexual abuse and battering.[1,21]

Every functioning community must resolve conflict beyond calling the police and turning the problem over to the state, and a healthy community is the best antidote against crime. Restorative and transformative methods seek dignified resolution of problems in the context of community, where, often with a facilitator or passing a talking stick around the circle, every interested party has a voice in coming to a resolution on which everyone can agree. Power imbalances must be taken into account. The experience, when successful, is empowering to the victim and humbling to the person who must assume accountability, offer restitution and reparation, and make a contract to work on rehabilitating herself. A community by definition shares common values, and conflict activates reassessment of the values by which their coherence is realized. A healthy community will ensure that resources are provided for the healing of both the person who was hurt and the person who caused harm. Healing is about solving problems and preventing their recurrence.

The goal of prison abolition is a logical step in the building of a civilization.[22-27] If someone presents a danger to others, they must be constrained for others' protection, but not in prisons as we know them. It is self-defeating as a society to invest not only billions of dollars but also our confidence in an institution that has not served its purported functions and that causes infinitely more harm than it repairs.

A healthy prison is an oxymoron. Whereas prison practices are punitive, negative and destructive by design, transformative approaches are nurturing, positive and constructive. It is a matter of ideology – retribution vs healing and reconciliation.[20,28,29] Restorative practices de-center punishment, seeking instead to make things right for all concerned, to offer restitution and make peace. Informal conflict resolution is an everyday experience in most communities, including those most vulnerable to social injustices. Most offenses occur between people known to one another, and are resolved between the parties affected. Often this includes informal intervention or counsel from neighbors, friends and family who want the relationship to be repaired.

The physical, emotional and mental harms that accrue within most prisons for women are straightforward human rights abuses, and do nothing to prevent crime, to deter or rehabilitate lawbreakers, or to compensate or heal the victim. The growing recognition of the value of restorative justice practices and the ideals of transformative justice offers new ways to think about the kind of society we want to inhabit.

## SUMMARY

Prisons damage a great many people at great cost and they lower the level of a nation's civility. The poor health that is generated by prisons reflects a society that allocates health care only to those who can afford it. The media generate fear of crime even as crime rates are declining, and a need for institutions of confinement and punishment is something the majority take for granted. However, prisons are not inevitable. They are a choice.[30]

## REFERENCES

1  Faith K. *Unruly Women: the politics of confinement and resistance.* Vancouver, BC: Press Gang Publishers; 1993.
2  Faith K, Near A, editors. *13 Women: parables from prison.* Vancouver, BC: Douglas & McIntyre; 2006.
3  Glick R, Neto VV. *National Study of Women's Correctional Programs.* Washington, DC: Law Enforcement and Administration; 1975–76.
4  Gordon AF. Globalism and the prison industrial complex: an interview with Angela Davis. *Race and Class.* 1999; **40**: 145–57.
5  Sudbury J, editor. *Global Lockdown: race, gender, and the prison-industrial complex.* New York, NY: Routledge; 2005.
6  Willmott D, van Olphen J. Challenging the health impacts of incarceration: the role for community health workers. *Californian J Health Promot.* 2005; **3**(2): 38–48.
7  United Nations. *Human Rights and Prisons: international human rights standards for prison officials.* New York, NY and Geneva: Office of the United Nations High Commissioner for Human Rights; 2005.
8  Canadian Association of Elizabeth Fry Societies (CAEFS). *CAEFS' Response to the*

*Canadian Human Rights Commission's Consultation Paper for the Special Report on the Situation of Federally Sentenced Women.* Ottawa, ON: CAEFS; 2003.

9 Campbell A. *Double Incarceration: maximum security in Canada's federal women's prisons.* Available at: www.prisonjustice.ca/politics/maximum_security_article.pdf (accessed May 25, 2009).

10 Schlanger M. Inmate litigation. *Harv Law Rev.* 2003; **116**: 1555–704.

11 Pate K. CSC and the 2 percent solution: the P4W Inquiry. *Canadian Women Studies Journal.* 1999; **19**: 145–53.

12 Arbour L. *Commission of Inquiry into Certain Events at the Prison for Women in Kingston: Arbour Report.* Ottawa, ON: Public Works and Government Services Canada; 1996.

13 Strupp H, Willmott D. *Dignity Denied: the price of imprisoning older women in California.* San Francisco, CA: Legal Services for Prisoners with Children; 2005. Available at: www.prisonerswithchildren.org/pubs/dignity.pdf (accessed May 25, 2009).

14 Hannah-Moffat K. *Punishment in Disguise: penal governance and federal imprisonment of women in Canada.* Toronto, ON: University of Toronto Press; 2001.

15 Hannah-Moffat K, Shaw M, editors. *An Ideal Prison? Critical essays on women's imprisonment in Canada.* Halifax, NS: Fernwood Publishing; 2000.

16 Cook S, Davies S, editors. *Harsh Punishment: international experiences of women's imprisonment.* Boston, MA: Northeastern University Press; 1999.

17 Comack E. *Women in Trouble.* Halifax, NS: Fernwood Publishing; 1996.

18 Boyd S, Faith K. Women, illegal drugs and prison: views from Canada. *Int J Drug Policy.* 1999; **10**: 195–207.

19 Skelton C. Ex-Mayors support injection site. *Vancouver Sun.* August 21, 2006.

20 Elliott E, Faith K. *Restorative Justice.* Burnaby, BC: Simon Fraser University; 2005.

21 Task Force on Federally Sentenced Women (TFFSW). *Creating Choices.* Ottawa, ON: Solicitor General; 1990.

22 Horii G. The politicization of imprisonment. In: Faith K, Near A, editors. *13 Women: parables from prison.* Vancouver, BC: Douglas & McIntyre; 2006. pp. 309–37.

23 Davis AY. *Are Prisons Obsolete?* New York, NY: Seven Stories Press; 2003.

24 Faith K. Seeking transformative justice for women: views from Canada. *J Inter Women's Studies.* 2000; **2**(1). Available at: www.bridgew.edu/SoAS/jiws/nov00/seeking.htm (accessed May 25, 2009).

25 Elliott L, Morris R. Behind prison doors. In: Adelberg E, Currie C, editors. *Too Few to Count: Canadian women in conflict with the law.* Vancouver, BC: Press Gang Publishers; 1987. pp. 145–62.

26 Culhane C. *Barred from Prison: a personal account.* Vancouver, BC: Pulp Press; 1979.

27 Culhane C. *Still Barred from Prison: social injustice in Canada.* Montreal, QC: Black Rose Books; 1985.

28 Morris R. *Stories of Transformative Justice.* Toronto, ON: Canadian Scholars' Press; 2001.

29 Elliott E. From scales to circles: restorative justice as peacemaking and social justice. In: Roberts JF, Grossman MG, editors. *Criminal Justice in Canada: a reader.* Scarborough, ON: Nelson; 2004. pp. 289–301.

30 Pate K. *Prisons: the latest solution to homelessness, poverty and mental illness.* WomenSpeak Series. Calgary. September 18, 2003. Available at: www.elizabethfry.ca/confernc/prison/1.htm (accessed February 23, 2009).

# CHAPTER 8

# Achieving Sustainable Improvement in the Health of Women in Prisons: The Approach of the WHO Health in Prisons Project

Alex Gatherer, Lars Møller and Paul Hayton

For too long now, the special needs of women in prison have received little consideration. The reason for this continued neglect, too glibly put forward, is the fact that women constitute a small minority of prison populations, and prison regimes have to be based on the needs of the clear majority of prisoners, namely men.

But this does not excuse the ignoring of important facts about women prisoners, namely that they have very different characteristics and significantly different needs; from society's point of view, a large majority of them have one or more children under 16 years of age for whom they are the primary carer. The imprisonment of mothers, usually at some distance from their homes, can lead to suffering in the children and to the breakdown of family relationships that have fundamental importance to societies. It is no longer justifiable to dismiss the special requirements of women prisoners as unimportant because of their status as a minority group. As most European countries confine pro-portionately more and more women in prison, it is urgent that action be taken so that their different and extra needs can be addressed. Most women are put into prison for using drugs or for drug-related crime. Many are drug-dependent and should, therefore, be considered for treatment rather than a sentence of imprisonment.

From the public health point of view, one of the most urgent tasks is to improve the health, resilience, and well-being of all those in compulsory deten-tion, and especially women. This is needed in their interests, in the interests of any family and social support roles they have, but also because of their import-ance to public health as a whole.

Despite all the difficulties of protecting and promoting health in the usually adverse environments presented by prisons, experience over a decade or so in Europe has shown that prisons, used as a last resort, can nevertheless be made into a setting in which useful health protection and promotion work can occur. Prisons can provide treatment and harm reduction measures efficiently and effectively and they can be used to provide help to some of the most disadvan-taged and hard-to-reach people in any society.[1]

This chapter outlines how a particular approach to supporting health care and health promotion in prisons has been developed in Europe – the WHO Health in Prisons Project (HIPP). This chapter will examine how HIPP has made sustainable progress in the health of women prisoners possible. The WHO Health in Prisons Project is a way of: (a) reviewing and changing policies relating to all aspects of health in prison; (b) collecting and exchanging experiences; and (c) highlighting and disseminating examples of best practice.

## THE WHO HEALTH IN PRISONS PROJECT (WHO HIPP)

It has long been recognized in health promotion that two of the most difficult and continuing challenges are, first, to reach those in greatest need and, second, to achieve sustainable improvement in their health. The WHO network for prison and health believes that its approach offers valuable opportunities to do both of these and to contribute in a worthwhile way to the public health in general.

The WHO Regional Office for Europe developed an important approach to the global aim of Health for All. Following the paradigm shift in health promotion that followed the dissemination of the Ottawa Charter,[2] there was an enthusiastic development of the settings approach to promoting health. This was based on the simple realization that health was intricately associated with factors in everyday living, and that better health could come from using the strengths of the settings to encourage healthy choices and allowing choice through healthy policies.

While it was felt that prisons could not be taken as a setting of everyday life, WHO accepted the recommendation of some eight countries in Europe that the concept of a settings approach should be tested out in prisons. Strong factors in support were the realization that the public health importance of health in prisons was being neglected throughout Europe and that, although problems in prison health were very similar in all countries, there was no mechanism for exchanging experiences on what worked well in tackling the issues. This was despite the very real public health problems that were being reported from all countries, such as the disproportionately high prevalence of HIV infection in prison populations, and the huge challenges of drug addiction and mental health problems in prisons.

WHO launched its Health in Prisons Project in 1995 with eight countries involved. There has been a rapid increase in the number of WHO member states committed to the Project and the network of nations now consists of 35 from all parts of Europe. An account of the history of the first decade, its achievements and the persistent barriers has been published.[3]

Whether or not the Project has made significant improvements in the health of prisoners, there is no doubt that it has uncovered a strongly felt need in the countries of Europe for a way of learning from each other about the best way to deal with what are seen as common problems of public health importance. The structure, organization and approach, developed over a decade and outlined here, may be of interest to other parts of the world.

## CHARACTERISTICS OF THE WHO HIPP

From the very beginning of the Project, it was felt that sustainable change and improvement would be more likely to result if those involved were senior people at a policy-making level in the government department responsible for prison health. The structure of the Project, therefore, required commitment at government levels; all member state representatives in the Project were selected by the ministry responsible for prison health, usually the ministry of justice in close collaboration with the ministry of health. In this way, the consensus recommendations of HIPP were based not only on best evidence but also on the experiences of member states as well. This important Project support at government levels was emphasized by another network characteristic. For the first time in the experience of the WHO Regional Office for Europe, the WHO Collaborating Centre for HIPP was based in a central government department, namely the Department of Health in London.

The Project works through a series of annual meetings to which usually a one-day conference is attached. These meetings are hosted by one of the member states involved in the Project, with other support from partner organizations such as the Council of Europe, the European Commission, the United Nations Office on Drugs and Crime and several non-governmental organizations (NGOs). The cost of attendance is covered by the countries themselves, wherever possible. The conference is used to consider in depth the draft statements prepared for adoption by the members, and the network meeting comprises reports from the countries themselves on current issues and on progress being made in the implementation of HIPP recommendations.

## VALUES AND GUIDING PRINCIPLES

Since its launch, WHO HIPP has clarified the values and principles underlying its aims and objectives. It starts with one of the most important fundamental values of society, namely respect for the inherent dignity of all human beings, whatever their personal or social status. These values support the basic aim of the Project, which is to assist those responsible for prisons in the provision of decent and humane service that includes quality health care and health promotion. WHO HIPP believes that this aim can best be achieved through working within an ethical and human rights framework.[4] One of the HIPP partners, the International Centre for Prison Studies (ICPS), has assisted the Project through its concentration on human rights and prison work. This Centre is based in King's College, London University; it aims to assist governments and other relevant agencies to develop appropriate policies on prisons and the use of imprisonment. Its influential publications include *International Profile of Women's Prisons*.[5]

From human rights comes the principle of equivalence. The health care available in prisons should be broadly the same in extent and quality as that available in the local community. This is not only a fundamental requirement of human rights but has also considerable public health importance. Many diseases that are a threat to public health can only be tackled by adopting strategies of prevention, control and continuity of care for all at risk, including those often disadvantaged inmates of prisons.

There is also an important principle of appropriateness; those deprived of their liberty by a court of law should be held in premises that are acceptable in terms of shelter, sanitation, ventilation, and warmth and that are suitable for meeting their particular needs. It follows that those, for example, with very serious mental illness should not be admitted to prison but to a hospital or institution which can provide the specialist care required.

Health care in prisons is sometimes viewed as contrary to the main aims of the prison, such as security and control. The reality of trying to treat prisoners with complex health needs has to be seen against serious limitations in terms of the prison's facilities, its environment, and its legal and political mandate. To ensure that prisoners' health care entitlements are met requires dedicated and well-trained staff, and they in turn need support and recognition from politicians and the general public. Unfortunately, society is seldom as understanding of what prisons are trying to do as is deserved by those undertaking a difficult task on its behalf and in providing them with the necessary support.

Prisons should be seen as providing a public service, as they contribute to public safety by enforcing the sentences of society's courts of law. While security inevitably leads to prisons with high walls and some isolation within communities, rejection by society and a general failure to try to understand and appreciate the service provided creates problems in recruitment of staff, and erects barriers complicating the important role of prisons in helping the inmates toward a better, crime-free life.

The HIPP project is based on a whole-prison approach. It defines a "health promoting prison" as a place of compulsory detention in which the risks to health are reduced to a minimum; where essential prison duties such as the maintenance of security are undertaken in a caring atmosphere that recognizes the inherent dignity of all prisoners and their human rights; where health services are provided to the level and in a professional manner equivalent to what is provided in the country as a whole; and where a whole-prison approach to promoting health and welfare is the norm.[6]

## THE HEALTH ISSUES CONFRONTING PRISONS

At the launch meeting of HIPP in London in 1995, it became clear that all prison systems in Europe were facing the same health issues, although not necessarily in the same order of priority for action. These issues were:

➤ communicable diseases, especially HIV/AIDS, tuberculosis (TB), hepatitis and other sexually transmitted infections
➤ drug-related problems
➤ mental health problems.

The first strategic plan of HIPP was to produce a consensus statement on each of these, based on experiences in each member state and on best evidence from selected experts, together with recommendations on what seemed to work best in the prison environment.

As regards HIV/AIDS and TB, considerable work had already been done. In fact, one of the first WHO documents on health and prisons was the 1993 WHO Guidelines on HIV infection and AIDS in prisons.[7] At a meeting of HIPP and UNAIDS in 1998, it was concluded that a revision of these was not necessary but that few countries had really adapted the recommendations to suit their own position nor implemented the clear advice the guidelines contained. Further detailed work has been done by the several agencies and NGOs concerned, and the current position is summarized in *Health in Prisons: a WHO guide to the essentials in prison health*.[4]

TB and prisons had been the subject of considerable research in eastern Europe and the Russian Federation. An important conclusion from this work was that any national strategy for the control of TB must include a strategy for its control in prisons. Close cooperation with key bodies involved in the control and treatment of TB throughout Europe led to the publication of a status paper on prisons and TB.[8]

It took HIPP two to three years to look at drugs and prisons. With the cooperation of the Pompidou Group of the Council of Europe, a large conference was held in Berne in 2001 and this led to a consensus statement: *Prisons, Drugs and Society*.[9] It became clear, during the collecting of evidence and experience leading up to the statement, that drug use is one of the main problems facing prison services in Europe. But it was also clearly demonstrated that much could be done within prisons in terms of detoxification, treatment, and prevention of the spread of blood-borne infections including HIV. Some aspects of harm reduction, especially needle and syringe exchange programs, remain controversial as far as prisons are concerned, although they are widespread in communities throughout Europe and evidence for their effectiveness and safety in prisons is substantial.[10]

It was felt that an even clearer declaration of the need for action was required, and so WHO HIPP in 2005 published a status paper: *Prisons, Drugs and Harm Reduction*.[11] This paper included a definition of harm reduction as regards measures in prisons: "In public health relating to prisons, harm reduction describes a concept aiming to prevent or reduce negative health effects associated with certain types of behavior (such as drug injecting) and with imprisonment and overcrowding as well as adverse effects on mental health."[11] HIPP thus acknowledged the negative health effects that imprisonment can have: effects such as the impact on mental health; the risk of suicide and self-harm; the need to reduce the risk of fatal drug overdose on release; and the harm resulting from inappropriate imprisonment of people requiring facilities unavailable in prisons, especially in overcrowded prisons.

A pioneering consensus statement had been published by HIPP in 1999 titled *Mental Health Promotion in Prisons*.[12] This paper was developed with the help of a partner of HIPP, Mental Health Europe, and was the first (and probably remains the only) statement on mental health promotion in places of compulsory detention. Its opening statement remains true a decade later: "in the absence of positive counter-measures, deprivation of freedom is intrinsically bad for mental health, and imprisonment can potentially cause significant mental harm."[12(p.4)]

One of the innovations in this statement was the introduction of a checklist of points for prison managers to consider. The importance of governors/managers in creating the overall ethos of a prison was stressed; in fact the checklist started with the assertion that "a concept of care, positive expectation and respect should permeate all prisons."[12(p.4)] Without such a vision, prisons carry obvious dangers for the mental health of prisoners and of staff. It was recommended that prisons should assess and review their policies and procedures regularly, using the approaches outlined in the statement as a guide. The aim was to provide ways for the personal development of prisoners without them harming themselves or others; for this to happen, prisoners had to feel safe, be assisted toward insight into their own behavior and be treated with respect and positive expectations.

The framework for a review of policies and practices outlined in this statement is of general relevance and value. Based on experiences in all places of compulsory detention, the areas to be kept under review were:

➤ *reception*, as this can be a traumatic and frightening experience
➤ *induction*, so that from the start prisoners are aware of the regimes of the prison and of the help available to them
➤ *a clean environment*, as an uncared-for environment lowers self-esteem
➤ *a controlled environment*, with staff in control at all times, to minimize when possible the harmful effects of overcrowding, poor physical facilities, poor sanitation, and inclusion of anti-bullying strategies and support for the more vulnerable
➤ management arrangements such as to show good *support for prisoners*
➤ good management and staff relationships, which are crucial, based on *support for staff*
➤ the promotion of contact with families, friends and the outside community
➤ regimes that include *a range of activities* to enable prisoners to make best use of their time in prison
➤ regimes and approaches that also allow some *personal space and privacy* if at all possible, including an assurance that confidentiality is respected
➤ and finally, although difficult within the necessary constraints of a secure prison, the promotion of *individuality*, by offering some choice and some (albeit limited) empowerment of prisoners so that they can preserve some feeling of control over their lives.

The statement concentrated on mental health promotion because at that time HIPP felt that prisons throughout Europe were diverting all those with serious mental health problems to places capable of providing the specialist treatment and care necessary for such patients. However, at a general review of HIPP's progress (see later), it was clear that the actual position in prisons relating to mental health was very different and was a very serious and increasing problem. Prisons were becoming the receptacle for large numbers of people with mental health problems and serious addictions. HIPP realized that a much broader approach was necessary and that guidance was urgently needed to help staff to cope with the 70–80% of their inmates who suffered from some form of mental health or addiction problem. A background paper providing the evidence to support an urgent call for action was produced and the Trencin statement on prisons and mental health was launched in June 2008.[13]

## ASSESSMENT OF ACHIEVEMENTS AND GAPS

At its annual meeting in 2005 held in London to mark the tenth anniversary of the WHO HIPP, three questions were considered at the international conference and by the 25 member countries represented.

1 *Was the HIPP still necessary?* The unanimous conclusion of outside experts asked to comment was that the major problems were very likely to persist for most, if not all, of the next decade. The network of countries from all parts of Europe who were committed to HIPP had grown very quickly and, therefore, indicated a felt need; faced with very similar and serious public health problems, the exchange of experiences in trying to deal with these together with an assembly of evidence and expert opinion was very valuable to improving prison health's contribution to general public health. But tackling the crisis in mental health and prisons and the Project's silence about the sorry state of women in prisons had to be lead priorities.

2 *Was the approach used by the Project still the best way of making progress and retaining participation by countries from both the east as well as the west of Europe?* In supporting the methodology so far used, there was a firm call for the Project to raise the issues more loudly and to make a greater impact. Compared to the position at the launch of the Project, prison health was certainly higher on the political, health and public health agendas. But much remained to be done in Europe; in addition, it was pointed out that the issues were global in nature and the exchange of experiences should where possible be more global.

3 *Were there glaring omissions in the work so far undertaken?* There was a difference here between those countries with resources and a reasonable chance of continuing improvements and those countries with virtually nothing, and where resources for prisons were only provided by outside bodies, and on a single problem basis. But representatives of the latter countries felt strongly that only one network of countries, with all countries of Europe as members, was definitely the approach they wanted as they felt the learning opportunities were greater and more reciprocal.

Subjects for further action were: women in prisons; improving the care for those prisoners with mental health and addiction problems; mental health promotion for prisoners and staff and especially for women and young people. Special needs so far not sufficiently considered included prisoners with low educational and social skill abilities and the growing challenge of non-nationals (already about 20% of prison populations); and developing the role of prison health in reducing health inequalities, which was a high priority of health systems in Europe.

## THE NEW STRATEGIC PLAN

Three major achievements since the above review encouraged the development and acceptance of a new strategic plan.

First, in 2007, after several years of persistent endeavor, WHO published *Health in Prisons: a WHO guide to the essentials in prison health.*[4] Based on the experiences of many countries in Europe and the advice of experts, the guide outlines the steps prison systems should take to reduce the public health risks that arise from compulsory detention in often unhealthy situations, to provide health and general care for all prisoners in need and to promote the health of prisoners and staff.

The book grew from the realization that one of the strongest lessons from the end of the last century was that public health could no longer ignore prison health. The rise and rapid spread of HIV, AIDS and hepatitis C, the resurgence of other serious communicable diseases such as TB, and the increasing recognition that prisons were inappropriate receptacles for people with drug dependence and mental health problems have thrust prison health high on the public health agenda. Any national strategy for tackling these serious conditions requires the inclusion of a prison strategy because, at any one time, prisons contain a disproportionately high number of people at greatest risk.

The underlying general principles throughout the book are those based on human rights and on a whole-prison multidisciplinary approach; both are very necessary in order to build the caring and understanding ethos now considered essential in the treatment and care of those deprived of their freedom. It is therefore aimed at all those who work in prisons and also at those in policy-making positions who are so important in ensuring that management and staff of prisons have the respect and support necessary for their essential public service roles.

The second major achievement was the introduction of a best practice awards scheme, designed to draw attention to best practice examples at prison level and to reward the outstanding initiatives of staff in trying new and often imaginative ways to improve the health and well-being of prisoners. Already some 30 awards have been made, and these are building up a useful and practical information base of approaches tried and assessed in different countries.[1]

The third achievement was the launch of a prison health database.[14] The prison health database collects information about all European countries on certain prison health indicators. Although in its early stages, this will, for the first time in a region of the world, provide a way of "keeping a finger on the pulse" of prison health and give some measure of progress and of emerging problems on which HIPP and others can decide their priorities and action plans. There are several important partners in this development; mainly, the European Monitoring Centre for Drugs and Drug Addiction (EMCDDA), Wissenschaftliche Institut der Ärzte Deutschlands (WIAD) and the European Commission.

From the above-mentioned review of HIPP and a survey of member states' advice and opinions, the new strategic plan covering 2006 onwards will:

➤ continue its core commitments to annual meetings and related conferences, best practice awards, building a database, and the development of status papers and declarations on those issues considered to be of priority in prison and in public health

➤ have as immediate priorities mental health and prisons. A statement was published in 2008 – the Trencin statement on prisons and mental health[13] – and another statement on women's health and children in prisons to be published in 2009

➤ continue its work on alcohol and prisons

➤ collect evidence and expert advice on the valued place of prison health within health systems, especially as regards the health of the most disadvantaged and hard to reach in any society

➤ draw attention to the contribution that prison health can make to reducing health inequalities

➤ contribute more to the growing interest in the view that violence is not inevitable in modern society.

## KEY STEPS FOR SUCCESS

1 Political and professional leadership and supportive public opinion are essentials if sustainable progress is to be made.

2 Rhetoric about human rights and pleas for an ethos of dignity and decency in prisons has so far failed to make the dramatic progress now needed. Techniques of policy analysis, policy development and how best to get the advocacy that will lead to policy change are now required.

3 Ignorance about what prisons are trying to do is no excuse for public indifference and inaction. Professional staff have a great opportunity to lead public opinion by showing the benefits to all society from, for example, applying a gender sensitivity in the criminal justice system so that the social capital value of women and the true social cost of imprisoning most of the women coming before the courts is better understood. The result would be a policy of imprisonment as a last resort and a greater use of alternatives.

4 The public health case for action is so strong that the failure of public health associations to pay much more attention to the whole subject should be tackled.

5 In Europe, the WHO Health in Prisons Project has had some real success in getting countries to review their prison health policies and practices. But Europe is the only one of the six regions of WHO with such a network. It surely will not be too long before the global threats to public health arising from ignoring the focal points of disease that prisons have become are recognized.

## WOMEN, WOMEN'S HEALTH, WOMEN WITH CHILDREN, AND PRISONS: THE NEW PLAN

Although the special needs of women in prison were recognized soon after the Project was launched, HIPP first commented on the subject in 2001, in the consensus statement *Prisons, Drugs and Society.*[9] In a small section on women, the report pointed out that there was a more significant proportion of women in prison for drug-related offenses than was the case for men. HIPP policy was that women who misuse drugs had specific health care needs, particularly those who were also pregnant. It recommended practices that included:

➤ providing specialist advice on treatment of pregnant women who are using drugs
➤ providing appropriate health and social care for mothers and babies living together in prison and for imprisoned women's children if living in the community, including assessment and maintaining contact with their mother in prison, while putting the interests of the child as paramount
➤ providing education on relationships, sexual health and harm reduction for women in prisons.

HIPP also included a chapter on the special health requirements for female prisoners in *Health in Prison: a WHO guide to the essentials in prison health.*[4] It recognizes that female prisoners have complex health needs, including mental health problems, self-harm and suicidal behavior, substance use problems and needs relating to their reproductive health. As regards mental health, the size of the problem is alarming; for example, in England and Wales around 90% of women prisoners assessed in 2004 had a diagnosable mental disorder, substance use problem or both. The chapter also points out that women are 14 times more likely than men to harm themselves while in prison. The chapter contains advice on dealing with such issues in the prison environment.[15]

One of the important changes being introduced in the new strategic plan for WHO HIPP, adopted in 2006, is to consider the health issues facing prisons in a much wider context and not just concentrating on them within the prison environment. This reflects Europe's developing interest in the settings approach to health promotion with its emphasis on healthy public policies, and inclusion of the more recent idea of "health in all policies." It is of course accepted that there remain major health policies from the first plan that are far from fully implemented and where progress has been slow. It was, however, clear when looking at mental health that a wider approach was necessary; for example, schemes to divert the seriously mentally ill to appropriate clinical facilities instead of prison required guidance to the criminal justice system as a whole on health implications and not just to prison authorities. In addition, during 2007/8 WHO HIPP examined the subject of women, women with children, their health issues, and all parts of their involvement with the criminal justice system.[16]

The new plan, therefore, includes the intention during 2007/8 to look in a more comprehensive way at the whole subject of women and women with children, and the related health issues in all parts of their involvement with the criminal justice system.

The fact that the representatives who attend the WHO HIPP network meetings are usually senior people from ministries of justice, and involved in policy development, strengthens the hope that current policies will be reviewed and that consensus advice based on evidence, expert opinion and members' experiences of what works and what does not, will lead to changes and improvements.

## SUMMARY AND CONCLUSION: OUR VISION

HIPP has a dream, in which all societies ensure that their places of compulsory detention are run on the basis of full recognition of human rights. In such detention facilities, all professional staff recognize that their commitment is to the prisoner as patient and deserving of the same ethical practices as generally apply in health care. The dream also includes a media that leads societies to recognize that prisons are undertaking a public service on their behalf and that it is in their own self-interest to see that prisons prevent the preventable and treat the otherwise hard-to-reach people so prevalent in prisons.

In that dream, the neglect of the particular needs of women in all aspects of society will be a thing of the past and the lack of sensitive and humane care for any women still in prisons will no longer be a blot of shame on the face of public health.

## ACKNOWLEDGEMENTS

The WHO HIPP owes its success to the current participation of 35 countries of Europe and the skilled support of partner organizations.

The authors are grateful to Ms Brenda van den Bergh, Technical Officer of Country Policies and Systems, WHO Regional Office for Europe, for reading and advising on a draft of this chapter.

## REFERENCES

1 WHO Regional Office for Europe. *Strategic Objectives for the WHO Health in Prisons Project*. Copenhagen: WHO Regional Office for Europe; 2008. Available at: www. euro.who.int/prisons/20060508_1 (accessed May 25, 2009).

2 WHO Regional Office for Europe. *Ottawa Charter for Health Promotion, 1986*. Copenhagen: WHO Regional Office for Europe; 2006. Available at: www.who.int/ healthpromotion/conferences/previous/ottawa/en/ (accessed May 25, 2009).

3 Gatherer A, Møller L, Hayton P. The World Health Organization European Health

in Prisons Project after 10 years: persistent barriers and achievements. *Am J Public Health*. 2005; 95: 1696–700.

4 Møller L, Stöver H, Jürgens R, *et al.*, editors. *Health in Prisons: a WHO guide to the essentials in prison health*. Copenhagen: WHO Regional Office for Europe; 2007. Available at: www.euro.who.int/document/e90174.pdf (accessed May 25, 2009).

5 International Centre for Prison Studies. *International Profile of Women's Prisons*. London: International Centre for Prison Studies, King's College. Available at: www.hmprisonservice.gov.uk/assets/documents/10003BB3womens_prisons_int_review_final_report.pdf (accessed May 25, 2009).

6 Hayton P. Protecting and promoting health in prisons: a settings approach. In: Møller L, Stöver H, Jürgens R, *et al.*, editors. *Health in Prisons: a WHO guide to the essentials in prison health*. Copenhagen: WHO Regional Office for Europe; 2007. Available at: www.euro.who.int/document/e90174.pdf (accessed February 27, 2009).

7 WHO. *WHO Guidelines on HIV Infection and AIDS in Prisons*. Geneva: World Health Organization; 1993. Available at: http://whqlibdoc.who.int/hq/1993/WHO_GPA_DIR_93.3.pdf (accessed February 27, 2009).

8 WHO Regional Office for Europe. *Status Paper on Prisons and Tuberculosis*. Copenhagen: WHO Regional Office for Europe; 2007. Available at: www.euro.who.int/document/e89906.pdf (accessed February 27, 2009).

9 WHO Regional Office for Europe. *Prisons, Drugs and Society*. Copenhagen: WHO Regional Office for Europe; 2001. Available at: www.euro.who.int/document/e81559.pdf (accessed February 27, 2009).

10 Canadian HIV/AIDS Legal Network. *Prison Needle Exchange: lessons from a comprehensive review of international evidence and experience*. 2nd ed. Toronto, ON: Canadian HIV/AIDS Legal Network; 2006. Available at: www.aidslaw.ca/publications/publicationsdocEN.php?ref=184 (accessed February 27, 2009).

11 WHO Regional Office for Europe. *Status Paper on Prisons, Drugs and Harm Reduction*. Copenhagen: WHO Regional Office for Europe; 2005. Available at: www.euro.who.int/document/e85877.pdf (accessed February 27, 2009).

12 WHO Regional Office for Europe. *Mental Health Promotion in Prisons: report on a WHO meeting*. Copenhagen: WHO Regional Office for Europe; 1999. Available at: www.euro.who.int/document/e64328.pdf (accessed February 27, 2009).

13 WHO Regional Office for Europe. *Trencin Statement on Prisons and Mental Health*. Copenhagen: WHO Regional Office for Europe; 2008. Available at: www.euro.who.int/document/e91402.pdf (accessed February 27, 2009).

14 WHO Regional Office for Europe. *Prison Health Database*. Copenhagen: WHO Regional Office for Europe. Available at: www.euro.who.int/prisons/20070221_1 (accessed February 27, 2009).

15 Palmer J. Special health requirements for female prisoners. In: Møller L, Stöver H, Jürgens R, *et al.*, editors. *Health in Prisons: a WHO guide to the essentials in prison health*. Copenhagen: WHO Regional Office for Europe; 2007. Available at: www.euro.who.int/document/e90174.pdf (accessed February 27, 2009).

16 World Health Organization Regional Office for Europe. *WHO Conference on Women's Health in Prison: correcting gender inequities in prison health*. Copenhagen: WHO Regional Office for Europe; 2008. Available at: www.euro.who.int/Document/HIPP/prison_gender_inequities.pdf (accessed June 30, 2009).

# CHAPTER 9

# Standards for Prison Health Care: US and British Approaches

## Nancy Stoller and Alex Gatherer

In this chapter, we examine accreditation, standards, monitoring, professionalization, and community-based care provision as means of improving prison health care. We use comparisons between the US and Britain to highlight the different approaches of the two countries.

## ACCREDITATION, STANDARDS OF CARE, MONITORING, AND PROFESSIONALIZATION

### The US Experience

The US has three categories of correctional institutions: one federal system, 50 state prison systems, and numerous city and county systems. Each is managed according to legislation, policy, and practice unique to the specific governmental unit. In addition, there is neither a national health service nor a universal health insurance program, nor is there routine use of local effective public health programs. While the federal prisons rely on staffing from the US Public Health Service, other correctional settings use a diverse mix of health service models.

### *Accreditation*

Since the mid-seventies, the US has experienced the emergence of national and state accreditation of prison health services, especially by the National Commission on Correctional Health Care (NCCHC). Founded in 1976 by the American Medical Association (AMA) and the American Correctional Association (ACA), the NCCHC has become the most important prison health accrediting organization and has accredited almost 500 jails and prisons. It hosts two major national meetings a year focused on accreditation methods and skills; trains and certifies correctional health care professionals (CHCPs); does policy and legislative work; and publishes a journal (*Journal of Correctional Health Care*) and a monthly newsletter (*CorrectCare*). These activities are designed to bring jail and prison health care in line with standards that are constitutional, appropriate, and congruent with community standards.[1]

Accreditation is a form of self-regulation, funded directly or indirectly by the institutions receiving it. Hospitals, universities, and professional schools use their accreditation to market themselves; this stamp of approval may be required for eligibility for public funding for everything from student loans to government contracts. Prisons and prison health services do not have to market themselves. They receive prisoners regardless of their quality. However, accreditation can be valuable for other reasons, such as helping recruit quality staff. In addition, the NCCHC claims that accreditation protects financial assets by protecting institutions from lawsuits.[2] If a prison is accredited by an organization with prestige, it can argue in court that it meets community or national standards in its policies and practices. Thus, the argument proceeds, it is clearly not violating constitutional standards of care. With regard to health services, NCCHC accreditation carries significantly more weight than accreditation by the ACA.

*Standards*

Any accreditation process requires that the applicant meet certain standards in terms of policy and practice. The NCCHC organizes its accreditation process through its *Standards for Health Services*.[3] The areas covered by the NCCHC Standards are: facility governance and administration; maintaining a safe and healthy environment; personnel and training; health care services support; inmate care and treatment; health promotion and disease prevention; special inmate needs and services; health records; and medical-legal issues.

The American Public Health Association,[4] through its Jail and Prison Health Task Force, has created its own *Standards for Health Services in Correctional Institutions*, which highlight public health concerns, including health promotion, violence prevention, environmental health, access to care, ethics, and human rights, in addition to the direct provision of medical care. While the APHA does not accredit correctional health services, its Standards are intended to serve as benchmarks of quality consistent with international standards of care and treatment of prisoners and respect for prisoner patients. It also emphasizes health care workers' roles as providers rather than custody personnel. The APHA, NCCHC, and ACA standards have been utilized in litigation, legislation, and criminal justice health care policy development as measures of minimum and/or humane standards for provision of health care in correctional settings. While standards provide guidelines, they do not carry an enforcement process. They are, therefore, primarily useful within a political, legislative, or policy process that inspires, creates, or requires their accomplishment.

### Monitoring

Within the US, monitoring is accomplished via legislative oversight committees and hearings, through administrative units with specific responsibility for corrections or correctional health, and by judicial means. Standing legislative oversight committees can affect budgeting for correctional environments and health services; they can also hold hearings to investigate charges of poor care or dangerous environments and can create new legislation when needed. Limitations of such committees include sporadic meetings and their legislative rather than administrative power. Consequently, they lack the resources necessary for visiting institutions to investigate daily conditions or enforce improvements.

Some states have oversight commissions. Key ingredients in effective administrative monitoring using an oversight commission include appointment of commissioners and staff on the basis of expertise; establishment of a schedule for monitoring; and implementation of sanctions and new policies when existing ones are lacking. While many states have oversight commissions, they vary widely in independence and power.

Successful litigation can result in a period of judicial monitoring to ensure implementation of court rulings. Judicial monitoring can last for years, and if court-ordered changes are not implemented, a receiver can be appointed. A receiver has the power to change hiring policies and recommend new facilities. Such a receivership was implemented in California in 2006 to improve the quality of health care in state prisons. This receivership goes further than monitoring by taking the responsibility for providing and improving care out of the hands of the corrections department and placing it within the federal court system. The value of a receivership is that it can be used to implement changes in a health care delivery system.[5]

A final type of monitoring found in the US is community-based monitoring, via non-governmental organizations. Many community organizations attempt to monitor conditions in jails and prisons, but few have access to the institutions themselves, with legal aid organizations having the most. Community advocacy organizations are independent from the work of the state, which is after all the basic source and engine of incarceration as a social practice. While the state and the courts may demonstrate ambivalence about prisoners' needs, prioritizing security over health, for example, community advocacy organizations provide a contrasting position, paying close attention to the physical, medical, emotional, or psychic harms that might be done to those who are incarcerated.

*Professionalization*

Prison health care employees are increasingly represented by unions and professional organizations such as the Academy of Correctional Health Professionals, the Society of Correctional Physicians, and the American Correctional Health Care Association. The impact of these memberships can be both subtle and profound: improving self-respect and connecting providers with appropriate continuing education that offers a perspective on ethics and community standards of care.

## The English Experience

The UK has three prison services; one each for England and Wales, Scotland, and Northern Ireland. This chapter considers only the position of England. England has one prison system and one National Health Service (NHS) that provides health care to all residents, whether they are outside or inside a prison. Since 1948, the government of the UK has carried a direct responsibility for the welfare of its citizens. Different mechanisms for carrying out that responsibility can exist, such as appointing agencies or quasi-autonomous bodies, but the highest proportion of the total cost of health services is carried by the state and the total amount made available is a political decision by the government of the day. A centralized management approach is, therefore, usual. The prison service in England is a national entity which for the past 40 years has been directly supervised by the Home Office, one of the major government departments of the UK. Management has been through the appointment of regional and area managers, and the aims and objectives laid out by the government. In England, it can be said that work in prison is truly a public service.[6] As will be seen later in this chapter, considerable involvement by the state in the provision of prison health services as with other public services in England has implications for the setting of standards and monitoring of the major government departments.

This approach reflects a marked level of state involvement. The government exercises a greater degree of central control over prisons than over other public services such as education and health and is held to account in Parliament, the legislative body, for the services provided, their extent and their standards. A high profile incident in any prison can be raised in Parliament and subjected to political debate. Accreditation is not, therefore, used and instead emphasis is placed on government setting the legal framework and the standards for an accountable managerial system to ensure compliance.

*Standards*

The prisons in England are regulated by national legislation. This means that an Act of Parliament lays down the broad principles (currently the Prison Act of 1952, with later amendments) and then the responsible department of government (the Home Office) issues Prison Rules, which are statutory instruments, namely secondary legislation. In addition, a large number of international covenants and treaties influence standards. The UK was fully involved in the development of these standards, which were accepted by government. Some of these are of central importance in determining how prisons should be run, and draw attention to the human rights of those deprived of their freedom by the courts. For example, the United Nations Standard Minimum Rules for the Treatment of Prisoners were agreed to as long ago as 1957.[7] Europe has also been influenced by the work of the Council of Europe that produced the European Prison Rules.[8]

In the late 1980s and early 1990s, all public services in England were involved in managerial changes aimed at making them more efficient and effective; if not businesses, at least more business-like. In 1993, the Prison Service was redefined as an agency of the Home Office and, for the first time, a Director-General was appointed who had a business background. He introduced a management approach similar to what was common in businesses. The Prison Service was given a Statement of Purpose, a vision, a set of six goals, and eight key performance indicators against which prisons were to be measured. These are updated regularly. The 2003 Statement of Purpose was: "Her Majesty's Prison Service serves the public by keeping in custody those committed by the courts. Our duty is to look after them with humanity and help them live law-abiding and useful lives in custody and after release."[9]

The Director-General reports to the Home Office and oversees a top-down management structure. The country is divided into several regions each with area managers who directly relate to the governors of individual prisons. Each governor is appointed with a clear contract stating responsibilities and reporting duties. They are accountable for the overall running of individual prisons; are expected to possess considerable leadership ability; and have a duty of care for prisoners in their charge, a concept with legal liability attached to it.

One difficulty with this type of approach is the inevitable growth in the number of performance indicators and key actions required. Managers may find it difficult to focus on all of them in their day to day work, making management accountability and monitoring essential to quality control.

One of the most important changes in the management approach occurred in 2004 with the creation of the National Offender Management Service (NOMS), an overarching body covering prisons and probation services. In January 2008, NOMS and the Prison Service were fully amalgamated; the chief executive of the restructured NOMS now runs public prisons and manages performance across the sector, through service level agreements and formal contracts with probation boards and trusts, and contracted out prisons. (Contracted out prisons are privately managed prisons, about 11 out of some 140 prisons in total.) The aim is to provide an "end to end" offender management strategy.[10]

*Monitoring*

The first step in monitoring a health care standard in England is through an audit procedure. Increasingly, throughout public services, the idea of clinical governance is expected to apply. Under this model, the physicians and nurses assess, improve, and maintain the quality of the service being provided. Audit systems are established as part of a quality assurance program.

In addition, the importance of establishing an open system in which the customer (prisoner, patient and relatives) can raise matters of concern, put in requests, and make complaints is stressed in public service management. Simple issues can usually be dealt with by the staff immediately involved. But there is easy recourse to a more formal procedure: a complaints form is completed and the senior staff decides how to deal with the matter. Both are documented and the finished forms become part of the manager's audit system. The prisoners can also ask for their complaints to be dealt with confidentially, and, if against the governor, can have confidential access to the area manager. In 1994, a Prisons Ombudsman post was created to look at complaints from prisoners about their treatment. Prisoners have the same right of access to the court and judicial review as other citizens. This includes applications to the European Court of Human Rights. Since 1998, when the UK Parliament enacted the Human Rights Act, which incorporated the European Convention on Human Rights into British law, prisoners can take up issues in domestic courts.

A well-established external monitoring arrangement exists in English prisons, and every prison has an Independent Monitoring Board. These volunteer groups have a direct interest in all matters concerning individual prisoners. Since 1981, there has also been an independent monitoring and inspection system under Her Majesty's Chief Inspector of Prisons.[11] This post reports directly to the Home Secretary, the most senior cabinet minister responsible for prisons. Prison inspection includes the right to visit all parts of a prison at any time, and reports go directly to the Home Secretary. This arrangement has been one of the most effective ways to hold closed institutions like prisons accountable.

The European Committee for the Prevention of Torture and Inhuman or Degrading Treatment or Punishment (CPT) independently monitors all places where people are deprived of their liberty in the member states of the Council of Europe. This committee is made up of a representative from each country involved, including the UK, but inspections are usually conducted by a small number of members with one or two experts. CPT reports are treated with respect throughout Europe, and although they begin as confidential, it is customary for the reports to be published along with the government's response.

A small number of privately run prisons have been built in England and are contracted out for management. The introduction of the marketplace into the prison service is the result of the government's reaction to the rising prison population and shortage of available places. The two types of prisons have similar external monitoring arrangements.

## PROVISION OF CARE BY OUTSIDE AGENCIES
### The US Experience

One approach to improving health care for prisoners has been to hire outside providers, such as public health departments, non-profit organizations, university health centers, or private, for-profit corporations. Some states have a mix of service providers. The use of outside service providers presents additional challenges for prison health care standards and accreditation. Private correctional health care vendors provide $3 billion of health care services annually to inmates in US correctional facilities.[12] Correctional Medical Services (CMS) currently serves over 250 000 prisoners at facilities in 24 states.[13] Monitoring private prison health care has proven to be even more difficult than monitoring the public system because the private firms have more freedom to provide their services without close scrutiny.

Private-for-profit providers also present a challenge for quality of care because one policy argument in their favor has been that they provide the same service as the public sector, but are more cost effective. The major saving is generally in staffing costs, with studies showing that private sector employees receive lower salaries and that up to 15% fewer staff members are used to deliver care.[14] Privately provided health services should be subject to public monitoring to guarantee that they are meeting the terms of their contracts.

Independent and academic medical centers also provide health services to prisons and jails and bring important advantages to these settings. Advantages can include: familiarity with current best practices; a primary identification with medicine instead of corrections; access to specialized training and continuing education, research skills and interests; and an ability to find specialists, clinics, and tertiary care that might be more difficult to access within a corrections institution.

Health departments provide services to prisoners in some cities and states. For example, in San Francisco, California, jail medical and mental health care is delivered by the county's Department of Public Health. The county's public hospital, San Francisco General Hospital and Medical Center, provides off-site care.

Despite accreditation efforts, newly promulgated standards, monitoring, increased professionalization of health care workers, and development of alternative providers, the last 30 years has seen a steady decline in the quality of daily life for US prisoners.

### The English Experience

Although the NHS was established in 1948, and included prisoners in its goal of health care for all, the provision of health care in prisons remained the responsibility of the prison service. In common with most of the rest of Europe, prison health was isolated from mainstream health services and the quality of care suffered because of difficulties in recruiting qualified staff.

In 1996, the Chief Inspector of Prisons in England drew national and political attention to the deficiencies of the prison health services in a report titled *Patient or Prisoner?*[15] This report made it clear that a new strategy for providing health care in prisons was required. In 2002, the decision was made to transfer the responsibility for health care in prisons to the NHS with a large financial investment. By 2006, the transfer was complete.

The situation in 2008 is that prison health is part of the NHS. Planning and purchasing health services are now the same for prisons as for the general community; prisoners use the same hospital and specialist services. As an example, prisoners have the same right to be considered for scarce organs for transplant as patients in the community; decisions are made based on clinical need and conditions, not whether the patient is a prisoner or not. The same expectations and standards apply to physicians and nurses who work in prisons as their peers in the NHS. They have the same conditions of service and salaries as others in the NHS.

Physicians working in the prison service can rightly claim the same professional independence as their colleagues working throughout the NHS. They practice within the European Prison Rules, and expect their management colleagues to respect their clinical independence. They expect full involvement with their local peers, including opportunities for professional refreshment, continuing education and inclusion in local medical affairs. They know that breaches of medical ethics will expose them to the same disciplinary measures as their colleagues in other parts of the NHS. Medical records belong to the NHS and the same requirements of confidentiality are followed. The same parity of professional conditions applies to other health care staff. Clinical errors made in prison are dealt with in exactly the same way as in general practice or hospital practice. (In the UK, general practice is the accepted term for the services provided by a general practitioner.) Prisoners have the same access to law in terms of clinical negligence and have their complaints dealt with in the same way.

It would appear that most of what is necessary to guarantee high quality health care in English prisons is available. In practice, problems and concerns remain. First, while there may be parity of professional terms and conditions, there is not yet parity of professional or public respect. It is still unpopular to work in the rather inhibiting atmosphere of prisons. Second, the tension between custodial and health care staff, with their very different aims, remains high and can lead to considerable stress. Third, real problems remain with access to secondary care, long recognized with prisoners with serious mental health problems, but also difficult in acute care including delivery suites for childbirth. But the merger of the prison health service with the NHS has continued a process of innovation and at least many of the glaring inadequacies and injustices of the not so distant past have been or are being tackled.

## SUMMARY AND CONCLUSION

The differences between the US and England demonstrate the significance of having one national correctional system instead of a fragmented collection of services, and the enormous importance of having a national health care system that can provide a prison health service with the same standard of care as is available in the community. As local and national jurisdictions look to policy change to improve prisoner health care, our review indicates that several simultaneous strategies may be needed. Improving care by applying standards is not enough, nor is simply bringing care in from outside the institution. Even when care in the prison clinic is equivalent to care outside the prison, as is the goal of the NHS experiment, there are insuperable limitations in the ability to "create health." Prison is a source of ill health and a locus of inevitable barriers and delays to health care access. While this chapter does not focus on the barriers, it is important to remember that they provide the starting point to the public health and medical argument for using imprisonment as a last resort and using alternatives to imprisonment wherever possible as the ultimate route to health for prisoners. Until then, it is surely not too much to expect that prison health services are not ignored or left isolated from mainstream health services and that attempts be made to ensure progress toward equivalent health care for those deprived of their freedom.

## ACKNOWLEDGEMENT

One of the authors, Alex Gatherer, would like to acknowledge the help of John Podmore in reading a draft relating to the English experience and advising on updating the management arrangements. John Podmore is a former prison governor and is Senior Operational Advisor to the Department of Offender Health, Department of Health, UK.

## REFERENCES

1 National Commission on Correctional Health Care. *About NCCHC*. Available at: www.ncchc.org/about/index.html (accessed February 28, 2009).
2 National Commission on Correctional Health Care. *Accreditation*. Available at: www.ncchc.org/accred/index.html (accessed February 28, 2009).

3 National Commission on Correctional Health Care. *NCCHC Standards.* Available at: www.ncchc.org/pubs/index.html (accessed February 28, 2009).

4 American Public Health Association. *Standards for Health Services in Correctional Institutions.* Washington, DC: APHA; 2003.

5 State of California. *California Prison Health Services.* 2009. Available at: www.cprinc.org (accessed June 19, 2009).

6 Coyle A. *Humanity in Prison: questions of definition and audit.* London: International Centre for Prison Studies, University of London; 2003.

7 United Nations. *Standard Minimum Rules for the Treatment of Prisoners.* Available at: www.unhchr.ch/html/menu3/b/h_comp34.htm (accessed February 28, 2009).

8 Council of Europe. *European Prison Rules.* Available at: www.uncjin.org/Laws/prisrul.htm (accessed February 28, 2009).

9 HM Prison Service. *Statement of Purpose.* Available at: www.hmprisonservice.gov.uk/abouttheservice/statementofpurpose (accessed February 28, 2009).

10 Podmore J. Personal communication. 2008.

11 Owers A. Independent inspection of prisons. In: Jones D, editor. *Humane Prisons.* Oxford: Radcliffe Publishing; 2006. pp. 177–90.

12 Mellow J, Greifinger RB. Successful reentry: the perspective of private correctional health care providers. *J Urban Health.* 2007; **84**(1): 85–98.

13 Correctional Medical Services. *Changing the Face of Correctional Healthcare.* 2009. Available at: www.cmsstl.com (accessed June 19, 2009).

14 Austin J, Irwin J. *It's About Time: America's imprisonment binge.* 3rd ed. Independence, KY: Wadsworth; 2001.

15 HM Inspectorate of Prisons for England and Wales. *Patient or Prisoner? A new strategy for health care in prisons.* London: Home Office; 1996.

# CHAPTER 10

# Ethics for Health Care Providers: Codes as Guidance for Practice in Prisons

### Janet Storch and Cindy Peternelj-Taylor

While recognizing prisons as unhealthy and detrimental places for all people, health care providers, including nurses, social workers, physicians, and others, can do a great deal to offer respectful health promoting care, to protect prisoners from research abuse, and to advocate for alternatives to imprisonment. In doing so, health care providers exercise their moral agency as practitioners, researchers, and advocates for appropriate health care and health-related research.

One means to accomplish these goals is through greater practical use of codes of professional ethics. Codes provide valuable directives for health care providers and enhance ethical reflection on complex problems. While codes alone are insufficient in promoting ethical practice, they can offer valuable guidance and serve as a platform for ethics education and dialogue. In this chapter, we borrow extensively from the Canadian Nurses Association (CNA) Code of Ethics for Registered Nurses.[1] We suggest that codes of ethics can guide and direct health providers' attitudes and actions toward greater alignment with their responsibilities for all people in their care. The structures and processes of prisons that inhibit attention to ethical practice will be discussed throughout the chapter. The chapter concludes with an emphasis on the importance of ethical practice in prisons, despite and because of the challenges of exercising one's moral agency within the prison environment. By moral agency we mean the capacity or power to direct one's motives and actions toward an ethical end, doing what is good and right.[1]

## CONTEXT OF "CORRECTIONAL" SERVICES FOR WOMEN

Ethical practice necessitates attention to context,[2] including the structures and the goals of institutions, and the manner in which those goals are or are not realized. Prison systems vary by country; for example, in England and Wales prisons are centralized under one authority that allows for uniform standard setting. In the US, three types of adult detention facilities exist: federal and state prisons and county jails, with considerable variation across states in terms of conditions. In Australia, responsibility for prisons rests entirely with the state/territory; and Canada has two levels of prisons: individuals sentenced to two years less a day or less are generally incarcerated within provincial facilities, while those sentenced to two years or more are incarcerated within federal prisons.

In general, the provision of health care in Canada is a provincial responsibility. However, once individuals become federal prisoners, provision for their health care is transferred to Correctional Services Canada (CSC).[3] Responsibilities for prison health services are clearly stated under enabling legislation that specifies CSC provide each prisoner with "essential healthcare; reasonable access to non-essential mental healthcare that will contribute to the [prisoner's] rehabilitation and successful integration into the community," and this provision of health care must "conform to professionally accepted standards."[3(p.S9)] However, a comprehensive study of Canadian prisoners showed limited available information about their health status and a lack of infrastructure to address the core functions of a public health service.[3(p.S51)] Most instructive about this report was the absence of data about health-promoting behaviors, such as good nutrition, physical activity, ready access to and use of counselors, etc.

## ETHICS, CODES OF ETHICS AND PRISON HEALTH SERVICES

Health providers constitute an important resource for prisoners. But how might these health providers deal with the conflicts that arise between custody and care? Specifically, how can they deal with demands for organizational loyalty and keep the care of their patients as their prime responsibility?[4] Health care providers constantly face the competing tensions enmeshed in their collective duties to the prisoner who is their patient, their profession, the prison system which is their employer, and the community at large.[5] These conflicting loyalties between professional and employer values are especially problematic in the provision of prison health care.

### Ethics as a Means and an End

Conflicting loyalties contribute to the moral distress nurses and other health professionals experience when they know what ethically should be done but are unable to fulfill this obligation due to agency policy or other external requirements.[6-9] Over time, many nurses succumb to meeting their employer's requirements as their foremost duty, by failing to keep the person in their care as their primary focus of responsibility. The latter is an expectation of nurses established in codes of ethics since at least 1973.[10] This is a particular concern for nurses who work in prison, where understanding the referent groups, particularly correctional staff, and the power they wield, is essential.

In participatory action research, investigators found that more explicit use of ethics in practice assisted nurses to rediscover commitments and find ways to restore their professional and moral identity. An important part of this exercise involved open discussion about ethics and collegial support in enacting values in practice.[11] A starting point in many of these projects has been to revisit the CNA Code of Ethics as guidance for practice.

### The CNA Code of Ethics for Registered Nurses 2008

The CNA Code of Ethics for Registered Nurses 2008 will be used as an example that can provide guidance for practice. The current CNA Code was released in June 2008 after almost three years of intense review and revision.

The 2008 Code speaks to the moral agency of the nurse and is based upon seven primary values central to practice. These include: (1) providing safe, compassionate, competent and ethical care; (2) promoting health and well-being; (3) promoting and respecting informed decision-making; (4) preserving dignity; (5) maintaining privacy and confidentiality; (6) promoting justice; and (7) being accountable.[1(p.3)] A concise definition of these values is accompanied by a set of responsibility statements that provide examples in practice.

### Codes of Ethics and Health Providers Who Care for Prisoners

The first value, *safe, compassionate, competent and ethical care*, contains two statements of particular significance for those working in prison.

> Nurses engage in compassionate care through their speech and body language and through their efforts to understand and care about others' health-care needs.[1(Section,A.2)]

> Nurses build trustworthy relationships as the foundation of meaningful communication, recognizing that building these relationships involves a conscious effort. Such relationships are critical to understanding people's needs and concerns.[1(Section,A.3)]

Prisoners may not have experienced trusting relationships with health care professionals, and the prison climate does not facilitate trust. But building trust through relational ethics, that is, through a relationship of mutual respect, engagement, and attention to the environment,[12] can be a powerful transformative experience and requires that health professionals become aware of the oppression and dehumanization that occurs in prisons. All prison health care providers must educate themselves about prisons and the meaning of imprisonment for the individual.

The value of *promoting health and well-being* requires nurses to focus "first and foremost toward the health and well-being of the person, family or community in their care."[1(Section,B.1)] It further recognizes and respects the expertise of other health care professionals to maximize benefits for persons receiving care.[1(Section,B.3)]

Several statements in the Code[1] underscore the importance of nurses thinking broadly about organizational, social, economic, and political factors influencing health. Nurses are urged to participate in addressing these social justice issues; to recognize the need for a continuum of accessible services; and to work toward improved access to health care. While prisons present a unique milieu for health care delivery, professionals must be attentive to prisoners' needs.

*Promoting and respecting informed decision-making* involves helping persons to express their health needs and values, as well as helping them obtain information and services so they can make informed decisions. Responsibilities include being "sensitive to the inherent power differentials between care providers and those receiving care."[1(Section,C.5)] The prison climate restricts autonomy and does not facilitate independent decision-making. Promoting a person's right to be informed and to make decisions is likely to involve some of the most challenging work for prison health professionals. Hannah-Moffat[13] notes that incarceration results in the loss of rights and freedoms that makes it difficult for providers to engage in health-promoting practices.

*Preserving dignity* involves recognizing the intrinsic worth of each person and includes advocacy for respectful treatment of all. Such a value in prison health services should exist even when many aspects of prison life sacrifice dignity. Responsibility for preserving dignity includes respecting the physical privacy of persons when care is given, as well as intervening when others fail to do so. Women prisoners often suffer from lack of respect for their personal privacy and the privacy of their information. Many current practices occur by habit, custom or sheer convenience, and only some are warranted. Prison health providers need to reflect and act upon those situations that can and should be changed.

*Maintaining privacy and confidentiality* involves safeguarding personal, family and community information. Confidentiality is a long-standing ethical dictum with particular relevance for prison health services. Health care providers are bound to "intervene if others inappropriately access or disclose personal or health information of persons receiving care."[1(Section,E.10)] When they are legally required to disclose confidential information, they have an ethical responsibility to "disclose only the amount of information necessary for that purpose and inform only those necessary."[1(Section,E.4)] Confidentiality should not preclude the anonymous abstracting of information that provides the prison system with information about prisoners' health status. Prison administrators require these data to inform planning.

*Promoting justice* is described as upholding "principles of justice by safeguarding human rights, equity and fairness, and by promoting the public good."[1(Section,F)] Responsibility requires that health care providers "advocate for fair treatment and for fair distribution of resources for those in their care."[1(Section,F.4)] An example of a prison policy that creates dilemmas for Canadian prisoners is that "some women have requested a longer sentence to be housed in federal institutions" because only federal prisons offer certain programs and services. Also, some women believe that federal prisons allow them to be closer to home and to be eligible for an earlier release.[13(p.217)] Many advocates for prison reform decry a system that lacks alternatives to simply adding more time to a woman's prison sentence. The Code also requires that nurses maintain "awareness of major health concerns such as poverty, inadequate shelter, food insecurity, and violence" and that they "work . . . for social justice and . . . for laws, policies and procedures designed to bring about equity."[1(Section,PartsII,x)] Positive improvements in these health concerns can have an effect in preventing imprisonment of women and assisting them if they become prisoners.

Another critical responsibility statement for prison health service provision is the following:

> Nurses do not engage in any form of lying, punishment or torture or any form of unusual treatment or action that is inhumane or degrading. They refuse to be complicit in such behaviours. They intervene and report such behaviours.[1(Section,F.3)]

The importance of avoiding complicity cannot be overstated; yet, it can be most difficult to avoid. Health care providers may become accustomed to the punishing environment, failing to remember that they are dealing with fellow human beings.[15] In prison, nurses and other health professionals often choose not to see, hear, or intervene, for fear of disturbing the status quo, resulting in conflict and uneasiness between health care and corrections staff.[15] This is an example of going along to get along.[16] Although health care providers in all settings struggle with issues surrounding whistle-blowing, in prison such struggles are magnified because staff rely on each other for personal safety: a powerful deterrent to speaking up, even when it is the right thing to do.[17]

Part II of the CNA Code titled Ethical Endeavours[1] gives attention to issues of social justice that are relevant to the ethical treatment of women prisoners. The following clause is germane to this chapter:

> Nurses should endeavour as much as possible, individually and collectively, to advocate for and work toward eliminating social inequities by: . . . understanding that some groups in society are systematically disadvantaged, which leads to diminished health and well-being. Nurses work to improve the quality of lives of people who are part of the disadvantaged and/or vulnerable groups and communities, and they take action to overcome barriers to healthcare.[1(pp.20,21)]

That all health care providers are answerable for their practice is the substance of the final value, *being accountable*. Responsibility emphasizes the importance of honesty and integrity in all professional interactions. Prison health care is a somewhat uncharted field of practice for many. Moves toward enhanced education and credentialing programs for providers are important to prisoner health and well-being.

### RESEARCH AND RESEARCH ETHICS IN PRISONS

Research in prisons is an important means of providing insight into the issues contributing to imprisonment and to understanding health problems and services within prisons. However, numerous accounts of prisoner abuse have led to the development of ethical research guidelines, review of protocols by a properly constituted Research Ethics Board, and limited research in prisons.[18] Although some suggest that this gatekeeping role is necessary to protect a vulnerable population from further exploitation, Byrne[19] wonders if the pendulum regarding prisoner protection has swung too far. While research is going on inside prison walls, it is often research determined by the prison system and conducted by researchers who are of the system. Double agency, whereby employees of the prison who do research also fulfill another role, whether clinical, custodial, or administrative, raises ethical concerns. This dual role can impact subject recruitment, informed consent, data collection, and the right to withdraw from a study without repercussions or prejudice, leading to closed agendas and implementation of questionable outcomes.[20,21]

A balance must be struck between researchers' access to prisoners and prisoners' protection from exploitation and/or poorly developed research protocols. Health providers have a role in identifying relevant research questions, participating in studies, and ensuring that prisoners provide informed consent. Consent involves regular attention to prisoners' reaffirmation of their understanding of the project and their continued willingness to be involved.

### SUMMARY

This chapter underscores the role of health providers as moral agents in their work with prisoners. The context of prisons involves significant ethical challenges for nurses and other health providers. Ethics in this chapter is considered both a means and an end: it is the way health providers interact with prisoners/patients, and the goal of safe, compassionate, competent and ethical practice. The CNA Code of Ethics[1] can inform prison nursing practice. This is not to suggest that the unique realities of prisons do not make applications difficult, but it is to urge all nurses to stand with colleagues working in and out of prisons to advocate for change.

## REFERENCES

1 Canadian Nurses Association. *Code of Ethics for Registered Nurses*. Ottawa, ON: Canadian Nurses Association; 2008.

2 Rodney P, Pauly B, Burgess M. Our theoretical landscape: complementary approaches to health care ethics. In: Storch JL, Rodney P, Starzomski R, editors. *Toward a Moral Horizon: nursing ethics for leadership and practice.* Toronto, ON: Pearson Prentice Hall; 2004. pp. 77–97.

3 Canadian Public Health Association. A health care needs assessment of federal inmates in Canada. *Can J Public Health.* 2004; **95**(Suppl. 1): S1–S63.

4 Peternelj-Taylor C. Forensic psychiatric nursing: the paradox of custody and caring. *J Psychosoc Nurs Ment Health Serv.* 1999; **37**(9): 9–11.

5 Peternelj-Taylor CA, Johnson RL. Serving time: psychiatric mental health nursing in corrections. *J Psychosoc Nurs Ment Health Serv.* 1995; **33**(8): 12–19.

6 Austin W, Bergum V, Goldberg L. Unable to answer the call of our patients: mental health nurses' experience of moral distress. *Nurs Inq.* 2004; **10**(3): 177–83.

7 Corley MC, Minick P, Elswick RK, *et al.* Nurse moral distress and ethical work environment. *Nurs Ethics.* 2005; **12**(4): 381–90.

8 Hamric A. Moral distress in everyday ethics. *Nurs Outlook.* 2000; **48**(5): 199–201.

9 Hamric A. Bridging the gap between ethics and clinical practice. *Nurs Outlook.* 2002; **50**(5): 176–8.

10 International Council of Nurses. *ICN Code of Ethics for Nurses.* Geneva: International Council of Nurses; 1973.

11 Rodney P, Doane GH, Storch J, *et al.* Toward a safer moral climate. *Can Nurse.* 2006; **102**(8): 24–7.

12 Austin W. Relational ethics in forensic psychiatric settings. *J Psychosoc Nurs Ment Health Serv.* 2001; **39**(9): 12–17.

13 Hannah-Moffat K. Creating choices: reflecting on choices. In: Carlen P, editor. *Women and Punishment: the struggle for justice.* Portland, OR: Willan Publishing; 2002.

14 Wagner N. *Ethical Ambiguity: can one do the right thing in a wrong situation? The case of Machsomwatch.* Conference on Globalization and Nursing; 2006.

15 Blair P. Improving nursing practice in correctional settings. *J Nurs Law.* 2000; **7**(2): 19–30.

16 Corley MC, Goren S. The dark side of nursing: impact of stigmatizing responses on patients. *Sch Inq Nurs Pract.* 1998; **12**(2): 99–118; discussion 119–22.

17 Peternelj-Taylor C. Whistleblowing and boundary violations: exposing a colleague in the forensic milieu. *Nurs Ethics.* 2003; **10**(5): 526–37; discussion 537–40.

18 Hornblum AM. They were cheap and available: prisoners as research subjects in twentieth century America. *BMJ.* 1997; **315**(7120): 1437–41.

19 Byrne M. Conducting research as a visiting scientist in a women's prison. *J Prof Nurs.* 2005; **21**(4): 223–30.

20 Edwards M, Chalmers K. Double agency in clinical research. *Can J Nurs Res.* 2002; **34**(1): 131–42.

21 Peternelj-Taylor CA. Conceptualizing nursing research with offenders: another look at vulnerability. *Int J Law Psychiatry.* 2005; **28**(4): 348–59.

# CHAPTER 11

# Advocacy

## Donna Willmott

The medical officer shall report to the director whenever he considers that a prisoner's physical or mental health has been or will be injuriously affected by continued imprisonment or by any condition of imprisonment.

– UN Standard Minimum Rules for the Treatment of Prisoners[1]

The ICN Code of Ethics for Nurses affirms that nurses have a fundamental responsibility to promote health, to prevent illness, to restore health and to alleviate suffering to all people, including detainees and prisoners.

– International Council of Nurses[2]

Health professionals have an ethical obligation to advocate for their patients, but what does this mean in a correctional setting? This chapter explores specific ways that health professionals can fulfill this obligation through individual advocacy for their patients in jails and prisons, by supporting the efforts of prisoners to advocate for themselves, and by working with community-based organizations to ensure the rights and dignity of their prisoner-patients through public education and policy change.

The ability of correctional medical staff to advocate for their patients is often compromised due to the conflicting priorities in a setting where confinement, isolation and security goals override the health care needs of prisoners.[3] This chapter profiles examples of health professionals working collaboratively with incarcerated and formerly incarcerated women and their community-based advocates to defend the rights and dignity of women prisoners.

## ACE: NURSES AND PEER EDUCATORS WORKING TOGETHER

Twenty years ago, a group of incarcerated women at Bedford Hills Prison in New York, with the cooperation of the prison administration and the support of their medical staff, initiated a program – AIDS Counseling and Education (ACE) – that became a national model for HIV/AIDS peer education in prisons.[4] ACE was built on the well-documented understanding that peer education is one of the most effective means of reducing the spread of HIV, and successfully applied it to a prison setting – no small feat given the fact that prisons are designed almost exclusively for security and punishment.[4] The ACE program offers information and support for HIV-positive women, both through one-on-one counseling and ongoing support groups that address the many levels of stress that are part of living with HIV. Peer counselors also offer HIV/AIDS education classes for all prisoners in an effort to prevent the spread of the disease and challenge the stigma attached to being HIV-positive.[4]

The nurses at Bedford Hills have played a crucial role in the success of ACE. In an article reflecting on its 10-year history, the peer educators and nurses discuss the ways they were able to work together as a team to meet the challenges of the epidemic:

> An HIV/AIDS peer education and support program in a prison presents important opportunities for nurses to extend their impact, and peer programs will be strengthened by working closely with nurses. Nurses can play a role in health education by strengthening the capacity of health educators. When the ACE program first began, a nurse in the facility came to the early meetings when women were first learning about HIV. The nurse presented several workshops that educated the first peer educators about the nature of the immune system in the body and HIV disease . . . from this collaboration, the ACE peer educators are now a resource for other inmates about many health issues prevalent in the prison.
>
> Nurses working with those inmates providing peer support to people are able to create a bridge between the patient and their doctors. Inmate peer counselors live 24 hours a day with other inmates, and, therefore, are in touch with women whose medical or emotional needs relating to HIV develop or change. Nurses working with a peer counseling program can be contacted when an inmate needs help, has clinical questions, or needs an evaluation.[5]

Conversely, the nurses are able to refer their patients to ACE for peer education and support, thus offering them access to an ongoing network of support. The ACE program has created a model of collaboration between medical staff and prisoners that is highly unusual in a correctional setting. The peer educators poignantly describe the ways their joint work has changed the atmosphere at Bedford Hills:

Nurses, along with other employees of the facility, have participated in events that ACE developed that build a sense of community and support. Once a year we have an ACE Walkathon . . . prison administrators, security personnel, clinical staff, civilians, and inmates show their concern by sponsoring women who participate in the Walkathon. The ACE Memorial Quilt is displayed and a names ceremony is the finale of the day. At this time, hundreds of women form a human ribbon and for a brief moment, our pain, sorrow and hope become one.

Nurses sponsor women who are walking in the Walkathon, and sometimes walk in it themselves . . . When nurses participate in such peer-led events, it creates a link between the medical department and the inmates, furthering trust, communication, and medical support.[5]

The ACE program offers us a rich model in which nurses can function most effectively to provide care and support to their prisoner-patients. A setting that acknowledges the full humanity and agency of incarcerated women challenges the dominant penal ideology and creates conditions to optimize their health and well-being.

## DIGNITY DENIED: COMMUNITY-BASED PARTICIPATORY RESEARCH THROUGH BARS

Legal Services for Prisoners with Children (LSPC), a non-profit advocacy organization in California with a 30-year history of serving incarcerated women, offers another example of a successful collaboration between health professionals, incarcerated women, and their advocates. In collaboration with community geriatricians, LSPC investigated the conditions of confinement for older women in California's state prisons. This community-based participatory research project was designed to begin with the self-identified priorities of incarcerated women. Building on their knowledge and strength, the project promoted their participation and used existing social networks, both inside prison and out. Specific objectives of this investigation included examining the conditions of confinement for women prisoners over 55, identifying barriers to their health and safety, and developing strategies to improve their health and well-being.[6] In spite of the many challenges with communication and prison visiting, consistent efforts were made to maximize the involvement of prisoners in each phase of the project.

Once clients identified the concerns of elders in their midst as one of their highest priorities, a questionnaire was sent to women in the state system known to be 55 and over. More than one-third of the older female population in the state prison system responded to the questionnaire, and 18 agreed to participate in personal interviews to explore the issues in greater depth.[6]

After data were collected and analyzed with the assistance of geriatric medical consultants from the University of California, San Francisco, LSPC staff drafted the preliminary findings and sent the document to core organizers among the prisoners, who reviewed the draft and made appropriate changes. After months of revisions made through in-person interviews and correspondence, a report entitled *Dignity Denied: the price of imprisoning older women in California* was released to the public.[6]

The report documented the many ways in which prisons are unsafe for older people: assignment to top bunks, cells with no handrails, long waits in line to obtain medication, and prison rules that require them to drop to the ground for alarms.[6] There is no retirement age in California prisons, and many older persons are at risk of injury because of inappropriate job assignments.[6] Older women reported a pervasive fear of abuse, from both fellow prisoners and staff, and nearly half responded "yes" to questions that are indicators of depression.[6] Some of the most poignant responses came in answer to questions about the future. As one woman explained:

> [O]ne of the biggest problems that we fear is that [prison officials] forget us and they don't take care of us . . . As you get older, what are they going to do with us, stick us in some hospital and let us die somewhere? I don't think they know what to do with us . . .. Let us go somewhere . . . we have served enough time in here. We're no longer a threat to society, why are you holding us?[6]

The findings of the report led to two categories of recommendations: short-term recommendations to ameliorate the conditions of confinement faced by older prisoners, and measures to reduce the number of older prisoners. Recommendations to improve the lives of older prisoners included the following: establishing an "over 55" status affording older prisoners age-specific consideration and assistance regarding housing, programming, and activities of daily life; designating a certain number of cells within the general population housing units as "over 55" cells; and instituting a geriatric work policy that allows older prisoners discretion in terms of job placement and scheduling.[6]

Given the challenges to basic human rights and dignity for elders inherent in the prison system, the extremely high cost of incarcerating them (over twice that of younger prisoners), and their low risk to public safety (recidivism rates averaging less than 4%),[7] LSPC put the greatest emphasis on the need for alternatives to incarceration for elders. Recommendations include expanding California's Compassionate Release law to include older and disabled prisoners and establishing a home monitoring program for older prisoners to serve the remainder of their sentences on home confinement.[6]

The participation by older prisoners in the research and dissemination of the findings and recommendations in *Dignity Denied* gave them an opportunity to educate people in the community about the many ways incarceration puts elders at risk and diminishes their health. It also encouraged their own sense of entitlement to certain rights they have as elders. They began approaching the wardens in their prisons to request permission to meet as a group in order to discuss their concerns and bring their suggestions for improvement to the administration. Each of the three women's prisons in California now has a self-organized group of older prisoners.

The data obtained from the original questionnaire was analyzed specifically for information regarding the functional impairment of the respondents by one of the collaborating geriatricians. Those findings were published in the *Journal of the American Geriatrics Society*, thus amplifying the project's impact and reaching a wider audience of medical providers and policy makers.[8]

LSPC staff, along with family members of incarcerated seniors and formerly incarcerated women, held a series of meetings with prison administrators and legislators to advocate for the recommendations in *Dignity Denied*. They participate in the California Nurses Association Task Force on Correctional Nursing to raise awareness of the needs of older prisoners among nurses working in penal settings. Staff members have made presentations at several public health meetings and conferences on aging in order to build alliances with community-based organizations concerned with the rights of older persons but for whom older prisoners have been an invisible population.

## SISTERS INSIDE: ENVISIONING A DIFFERENT WORLD

One of the most notable advocacy organizations serving incarcerated women is Australia's Sisters Inside, founded by Debbie Kilroy, a former prisoner who, since her release, has committed herself to support the women inside. "We were not an organization coming in to the prison and trying to dictate to the women what they needed, what they wanted, what was wrong. From the very beginning, it was enshrined in our constitution that women inside were the decision makers. They constituted the steering committee . . . this is where we differ from many other prison advocacy organizations. The women inside are in charge."[9]

Sisters Inside has a long history of providing services to imprisoned and newly released women. Begun in the early 1990s, when Australia was in a period of prison reform, Sisters Inside was permitted to come into the prisons to offer essential services to women, such as sexual assault counseling and drug and alcohol counseling. The organization later developed transition support services and reconnection programs to preserve relationships between incarcerated mothers and their children.

In addition to providing services, Sisters Inside advocates for legal reform and policy changes affecting incarcerated women and their families. It has challenged the discrimination faced by women prisoners based on their gender, economic status, race and disability status.[10] It has advocated for the human rights of incarcerated women by waging a campaign against mandatory strip-searching, which traumatizes women, the vast majority of whom have been subject to physical, sexual and psychological violence much of their lives.[11] It has drawn attention to the racist nature of the prison system, which incarcerates indigenous women at a dramatically disproportionate rate.[10]

Perhaps most significantly, Sisters Inside educates the free world community about women in prison and raises critical questions about the efficacy of prisons as a way to achieve public safety.

> How can we say that prisons "work" when more than 60% of women who go to prison return to prison? That's an astounding failure rate. If we applied it to any major organization funded by the government, heads would roll.
>
> The prison experience is built on the twin lies of "community safety" and "rehabilitation." That first lie, community safety, seems laughable when the numbers of women imprisoned for violent crime is very low . . . and when we look at the effects of drug offenses and of long histories of continued sexual and physical abuse . . .. The second, rehabilitation? Without programs, without education, with the retraumatizing effects of strip-searching and detention in isolation? What do we expect?
>
> Do we really expect a woman whose life has been scarred by poverty and abuse and addiction, who is locked up, separated from her family, her children, any support she may have had, denied her human rights, denied the chance to gain any skills or training, humiliated constantly – do we really expect that when she is finally let out of prison she will be a better person? No money, no home, no job, no kids, and no self-esteem, but still a more effective member of the community?[9]

The ability of Sisters Inside to raise the overarching critical questions about the nature of the current criminal justice system at the same time it serves women incarcerated within it makes it a vital example of community-based advocacy for women prisoners.

## THE CANADIAN ASSOCIATION OF ELIZABETH FRY SOCIETIES

The Canadian Association of Elizabeth Fry Societies (CAEFS) is a federation of 26 local, community-based service providers who work with and on behalf of imprisoned women.[12] Their main goals are to promote decarceration for women, to reduce the numbers of women who are criminalized and imprisoned in Canada, and to increase the availability of community-based social services for marginalized and imprisoned women.[12]

In 2003, CAEFS filed a complaint with the Canadian Human Rights Commission on behalf of all women serving federal terms in Canada, charging systemic discriminatory treatment. Citing discrimination based on sex, race, and disability, CAEFS highlighted the particular conditions faced by Aboriginal women, mentally ill women and women segregated in maximum security units.[13] After years of public pressure, CAEFS won a major victory in June 2007, with the signing of a mediated agreement with Manitoba Province to address complaints about conditions of incarceration there. Under the agreement, women prisoners will have one-to-one counseling, improved spiritual services, a new program to facilitate access to their children, and women's advisory committees with consultation and input into services and programs.[14]

In addition to challenging conditions of confinement that violate the human rights of prisoners, much of CAEFS' advocacy is focused on encouraging the development of community-based alternatives to the enormous cost, both fiscal and social, of the over-reliance on incarceration.[15] In this, they share the underlying tenets of both Sisters Inside and LSPC's campaign for older prisoners, an understanding that the continued incarceration of huge numbers of women who pose little or no risk to the community does nothing to benefit the person who transgressed, the victim, or the community.

An important contribution of the Elizabeth Fry Society is Changing Paths, an innovative program developed from a feminist and learner-centered perspective for women in conflict with the law.[16] Instead of being incarcerated, women who have committed certain low-level offenses such as shoplifting, fraud, solicitation, or public drunkenness can be mandated by the court to Changing Paths. Changing Paths is predicated on an understanding that the majority of women who come to the program live in poverty, are subjected to violence, are struggling with poor health, both mental and physical, and have typically been silenced because of their marginalized status.[16] The program combines literacy skills and life skills:

> Literacy skills are the means for women to find their voice, grieve losses, celebrate success, advocate, heal, build self-esteem, and experience connectedness. Developing literacy skills is a way to build strength and capacity, and is a tool for personal empowerment . . . [it is] a springboard to naming, making meaning of, and taking action on life issues.[16]

Life skills include Aboriginal crafts, food preparation, computer skills, and "talking circles." This holistic approach combines intensive interior emotional work and intellectual work to help women heal at the same time as they develop their capacity to change those aspects of their lives that they want to change.[16]

## SUMMARY

Health professionals and other service providers who come into contact with incarcerated women or women newly released back into the community have an important role to play in defending their human rights and dignity. By working with imprisoned women in a spirit of collaboration, they can create innovative programs to address the needs of prisoners and former prisoners. By working together, health professionals, prisoners' rights advocates, prisoners, and former prisoners can encourage policy change that will lessen the negative impact of incarceration on the communities. Perhaps most importantly, these alliances can raise critical questions about the efficacy of prisons as the solution to our collective safety, and support alternatives to a strictly punitive criminal justice model in order to move closer to the kind of society we want to live in.

## REFERENCES

1 United Nations. *Standard Minimum Rules for the Treatment of Prisoners*. Available at: www.unhchr.ch/html/menu3/b/h_comp34.htm (accessed February 28, 2009).

2 International Council of Nurses. *Nurses' Role in the Care of Prisoners and Detainees: position statement of the International Council of Nurses*. 2005. Available at: www.icn.ch/PS_A13_NursesRole%20DetaineesPrisoners.pdf (accessed February 28, 2009).

3 Joint Nursing Practice Commission. Correctional nurses and collective patient advocacy: conclusions and recommendations from CNA's first Correctional Nursing Task Force. *California Nurse*. 2005; **101**(6): 38–9.

4 AIDS Counseling and Education Program (ACE). *Breaking the Walls of Silence: AIDS and women in a New York State maximum-security prison*. Woodstock, NY: Overlook Press; 1998.

5 Boudin K, Clark J, Flournoy V, *et al*. ACE: a peer education and counseling program meets the needs of incarcerated women with HIV/AIDS issues. *J Assoc Nurses AIDS Care*. 1999; **10**(6): 90–8.

6 Strupp H, Willmott D. *Dignity Denied: the price of imprisoning older women in California*. San Francisco, CA: Legal Services for Prisoners with Children; 2005. Available at: www.prisonerswithchildren.org/pubs/dignity.pdf (accessed February 28, 2009).

7 Aday R. *Aging Prisoners: crisis in American corrections*. Westport, CT: Praeger; 2002.

8 Williams B, Lindquist K, Sudore R, *et al*. Being old and doing time: functional impairment and adverse experiences of geriatric female prisoners. *J Am Geriatr Soc*. 2006; 54(4): 702–7.

9 Kilroy D. Australian community idol finalist speech. Available at: www.sistersinside.com.au/media/idolspeech.pdf (accessed February 28, 2009).

10 Sisters Inside. *Submission number 2: women in prison review: Anti-Discrimination Commission of Queensland*. Available at: www.sistersinside.com.au/media/submission2.pdf (accessed February 28, 2009).

11 Kilroy D. *Women in voice – women with voice*. James Cook University speech. Available at: www.sistersinside.com.au/media/womeninvoicespeech.pdf (accessed February 28, 2009).

12 Canadian Association of Elizabeth Fry Societies. *Goals.* Available at: www.elizabethfry .ca/egoals.html (accessed February 28, 2009).

13 Canadian Association of Elizabeth Fry Societies. *Submission to the Canadian human rights commission for the special report on the discrimination on the basis of sex, race and disability faced by federally sentenced women.* Available at: www.elizabethfry.ca/ submissn/specialr/1.htm (accessed February 28, 2009).

14 CBC News. *Human rights complaint leads to improvements for incarcerated women.* June 28, 2007. Available at: www.prisonjustice.ca/starkravenarticles/manitoba_ hrights_0707.html (accessed February 28, 2009).

15 Pate K. *Women in Corrections: the context, the challenges.* Proceedings of the Women in Corrections: Staff and Clients Conference. October 31–November 1, 2000. Adelaide, Australia.

16 Sochatsky B, Stewart S. *Changing Paths: a literacy and life skills program for women in conflict with the law.* Edmonton, AB; Elizabeth Fry Society of Edmonton; 2003. Available at: www.nald.ca/clr/changing/changing.pdf (accessed February 28, 2009).

# CHAPTER 12

# Teaching and Learning
# for Social Transformation

Judy Parker, Lisa Reynolds and Donna Willmott

In this chapter we bring together many of the issues that have been addressed in previous chapters and direct them toward the educational needs of professionals, policy makers, community workers and members of the public concerned about the health status of incarcerated women. We believe that education can play a crucial role in shifting attitudes and values. A plea is made for the importance of curricula that will broaden individuals' horizons and challenge stereotypical and negative ways of thinking about women in prison toward a recognition of the socio-political and structural reasons that lie behind their incarceration. It is hoped that by adopting an emancipatory approach to curricula development, impediments to health encountered by women in prison will be confronted and learners provided with tools that may be used to work toward improving the health and well-being of incarcerated women.

A social justice approach to teaching and learning is therefore highlighted and we draw upon ideas stemming from Paulo Freire in his famous work *The Pedagogy of the Oppressed*.[1] Many women who are prisoners and ex-prisoners feel profoundly disempowered by virtue of their life experiences. We believe it is important, wherever possible, that they are psychologically strengthened and a sense of hope and feeling of self-worth fostered through their dealings with health professionals and those working in or around the prison system. Therefore, education programs addressing health needs cannot be based on notions of health simply as absence of disease. Health needs to be thought of holistically, encompassing a sense of wholeness, well-being and interconnectedness at all levels: body and mind, family and community, with integration into relevant social organizations. Health problems experienced by women prisoners and ex-prisoners need to be addressed not only at the individual therapeutic level but also require an understanding of issues affecting health created by broader socio-political and economic issues of disadvantage, discrimination and poverty. This chapter is addressed to those who are interested in developing and implementing curricula around these ideas and within the value system that has been articulated so well by Freire.

## A SOCIAL JUSTICE APPROACH TO TEACHING AND LEARNING

Paolo Freire was involved in literacy campaigns among peasants in Brazil in the 1960s and developed a radical method of literacy education based upon the goal of liberation. While these ideas might today have a distinctly old-fashioned sound, the profound influence of his writings cannot be underestimated. He believed that the goal of liberation is to develop critical awareness, made possible through reflection and action upon the world, with the aim of transforming it. He argued that education aimed at liberation is based upon a democratic partnership between teacher and student, whereby each is both teacher and student. Teaching focuses around people's everyday lives and the imperatives of their local realities. Both the content and the democratic method of teaching are understood to inspire inquiry, creativity and critical thinking. He suggests that this method of teaching and learning, and the critical awareness that emerges from it, are integral to both ontology and epistemology: to being and to knowing.

Freire contrasted this mode of teaching and learning with what he described as "banking education," which separates the learner from the content and process of education. This educational approach assumes that the teacher is all knowing and the student an empty vessel into which knowledge is poured. Freire believed strongly that this form of information transfer becomes a symbol and an instrument of oppression, inhibiting openness to learning and new ways for thought and discussion. This is what he meant when he identified the teacher as oppressor and the student as oppressed. Both are part of the same system, each contributing to the maintenance of an oppressive relationship which inhibits open dialogue. Freire's message has withstood the test of time and remains extremely relevant today among progressive educators. Additionally, his commitment to unite theory with practice remains a lasting challenge to the field of critical adult education.[1]

## DESIGNING A CURRICULUM

When designing curricula within this educational philosophy, it is important that they are based on these fundamental principles of equality, inclusiveness and openness to new ideas. Curricula should therefore be developed not only out of the literature and the personal experiences of the educationalist, but all relevant stakeholders should also have a voice in their design, content, implementation and evaluation. For a curriculum to be developed to meet the learning needs of those involved either directly or indirectly in the health of women in prison, it would be appropriate for meetings to be held with key stakeholders to identify and elucidate issues that will inform the content.

These discussions are fundamentally important in that they provide the basis for ensuring not only that the voices of those involved are included, but they can also provide a means of ensuring that the content to be included in the curriculum is sensitive to local needs. For example, a curriculum that is designed for health workers in remote Aboriginal communities in Australia will have somewhat different priorities and imperatives from those of a curriculum designed for health workers in a large US city. Additionally, while the health issues faced by women in prison appear to be remarkably similar in many countries of the world, it is very important that underlying differences are brought to the surface. Criminal justice, health and welfare and education policies differ substantially between jurisdictions and curricula need to address local constraints and possibilities.

Those involved in discussions could include prison and community health care workers, doctors and nurses; prisoners and ex-prisoners; families of prisoners; community advocacy groups; and prison officers, guards and administrators. Group discussions would need to be conducted so as to ensure all views are canvassed and attended to. It would be important to ensure that health issues facing particular groups in prison are addressed: for example, pregnant women and issues surrounding childbirth, women with mental or physical disability, indigenous women, older women, and those with special health problems (e.g. diabetes, heart disease, etc.).

It can also be very useful for those developing curricula to be aware of differences in policies across jurisdictions. It can be extremely enlightening for participants in courses to be exposed to ideas that cause them to question some of their own taken for granted acceptance of various juridical constraints. Exposure to such ideas can help the development of a critical consciousness and the desire for social change. It is therefore important for those charged with the development and implementation of curricula to be linked to a wider international network to ensure ongoing exchange of ideas, innovations, enlightened policies, research and relevant literature.

## KEY CURRICULUM CONTENT ISSUES

There are a number of key topics that recur in the literature and in the experience of educators in this field. These need to be kept in mind when designing any curriculum, being mindful at all times that they need to be addressed in ways that ensure their relevance to local needs and to the specific requirements, wants and desires of course participants. These subjects aim not only to increase the understanding of participants about concerns surrounding the health status of women in prison, but also to encourage social change to occur that will enable improved access to health care by incarcerated women. These topics include the role of prisons in society; the culture of prisons and the impact of this upon the health of prisoners and upon those working within the system; the effect upon local communities of women's imprisonment; issues surrounding reentry to the community and advocacy for structural change.

## The Role of Prisons in Society

It is important that course participants can gain a broad understanding of the place of prisons in various societies and the specific populations that tend to become criminalized. This will facilitate understanding of the role prisons play in social control, and that those working in these settings are in fact agents of social control. Additionally, those who become criminalized can usually be identified in relation to categories of "race," gender, poverty, disadvantage and discrimination of various kinds. Prisons reflect systemic inequalities found in the wider society and participants could explore the ways in which prisons then tend to intensify these inequalities. It would be very illuminating for participants if prisoners and ex-prisoners or members of their families could be included as participants in discussions of this kind. The transformative/emancipatory potential of training/education is likely to be enhanced through the involvement of prisoners or family members throughout the development and delivery of curricula. However, prisoners involved in training must be supported and their safety ensured. Therefore it may be helpful to consider the use of information communication technology (ICT) for the development of reusable learning objects such as video clips and podcasts to safely incorporate prisoners' experiences of the prison system into learning activities.[2]

Consideration of these issues will help participants to gain a broader understanding of the societal structures that help to create and maintain both prisons and prisoners. An analysis of deinstitutionalization policies that have been implemented in many countries over recent years, for example in relation to developmental disability and mental illness, may point the way to possibilities for change in relation to the criminal justice system. However, the problem with these policies has been the failure of governments to provide adequate community support for those people and many now end up in prison, resulting in institutionalization of a worse kind. Discussion around the role of prisons could lead to consideration of whether they should be abolished and replaced with community programs.

## The Culture of Prisons and the Impact Upon the Health of Prisoners and Upon Those Working Within the System

The prison is marginalized from the wider community and its culture reflects this separation. Prisoners are thus doubly disadvantaged. Most are already members of marginalized communities and they are placed in a context which itself is divorced from the wider community. This sets up the preconditions for oppressive relationships and violence and works against efforts designed to facilitate therapeutic relationships and interactions based on a sense of equality. Participants need to gain an understanding of how the toxic culture of incarceration impacts on the health of women in prison.

The disruption to family life, dislocation from family, friends and community and consequent loss of loved ones can exacerbate illicit drug use, self-inflicted injuries, guilt, grief, despair and even lead to suicide. Additionally, women in prison are more likely than those in the general community to suffer from infectious diseases, respiratory conditions, sexually transmitted diseases, mental health problems, substance withdrawal, and be subjected to violence and injury. They can be exposed to infectious diseases, such as tuberculosis, HIV, and hepatitis C, and receive a poor diet and substandard medical care. If they have been substance abusers, or if they suffer from mental illness, they may not be able to have appropriate treatment, and they may suffer violence and injury. The curriculum could therefore include content that explores possible roles for frontline health workers in mitigating the negative consequences of imprisonment on those they serve.

Nevertheless, it is also important for participants to recognize the strengths of women in prison who work within their circumstances to survive, support and teach each other. Course participants need to learn about the models of peer education (e.g. in HIV, drug and childcare education) that have been extremely effective. This is a very important understanding for participants to gain so that they may be disabused of any ideas they have about adopting a "banking" model of education when in teaching and learning relationships with prisoners. Peer education is the optimal tool for promoting health in the unhealthy prison environment and participants need to consider means of encouraging such programs.

Discussion of issues around the negative effects of imprisonment upon health can plant the seeds for some initial discussion about the appropriateness of prison for women whose health is already compromised. The idea of public health and medical professionals being involved in developing community-based models enables the issue of incarceration to be considered as a health issue, not simply a criminal justice issue. Such an understanding is critical to developing awareness of the destructive impact of prison upon already vulnerable people and the need for a major shift in thinking that could lead to community-based models of harm reduction and prevention that are based on treatment not punishment.

### The Effect of Women's Imprisonment Upon Local Communities

Local communities can be severely disrupted when key members who may have had responsibility for children and for holding a family together are severed from their local connections. Families can be fractured, parental rights lost, and the emotional and social effect on children can be devastating. Burdens upon grandmothers caring for children whose mothers are in prison can weigh them down with responsibilities and tasks they feel ill equipped to cope with. It is important that the curriculum is developed so as to provide a means of opening a dialogue between the prison and the community. One way of approaching this could be to involve various agencies in the development of this aspect of the curriculum. The needs of women in prison are complex and are impacted by many different individuals, agencies and organizations operating both inside and outside the prison system. Therefore it is important that women prisoners, their families and the wide range of service providers involved with women prisoners and their families are consulted.

Furthermore, it would be useful to design curricula for inter-professional/ inter-agency learning in order to encourage cross boundary working, effective communication and joint policy development.

### Issues Surrounding Reentry to the Community

The issue of how education programs can be utilized to reengage prisoners with society is very important, as there are multiple systemic barriers to reentry to the community in many jurisdictions. Women have to rebuild family relationships, seek employment, education and health care. Since course participants may not be working in prisons or jails, but may be seeing former prisoners in the community setting, it is important for them to understand the complex issues women may face. In the US, for example, post-conviction penalties are staggering: people with a drug felony conviction may be denied welfare and food stamps for the remainder of their lives; they are denied access to federally subsidized housing; job applications are commonly required to state if the applicant has ever been convicted of a felony; and several job categories require background checks on all applicants.

### Advocacy for Structural Change

Course developers and course participants may each have very different ideas about the type and level of change they wish to advocate for. This can be an important area of discussion in class. Those advocating abolition of prisons and the provision of community-based models that manage the custody/care issues very differently from prisons can engage in healthy debate with those who might take a more conservative approach to change. If there are health professionals, such as physicians and nurses, in the class, the importance of their work in developing harm reduction/preventive models based on treatment rather than punishment cannot be overemphasized.

An important discussion is that of considering models of prevention aimed at, for example, decreasing gang violence and childhood abuse and increasing drug treatment programs. Discussion and debate can focus on current criminal justice, health and welfare policies and the extent to which community-based alternatives to incarceration can be promoted in the local area of interest. Questions can be raised about the possibility of restorative justice. The role of community-based health workers in organizing for change can be discussed, particularly in the area of overcoming systemic barriers to entry to the community. Best practices internationally can be considered and the feasibility of implementing them locally considered. These might include peer counseling training and meeting physical needs, resources available to prisoners, centers for prisoner education, peer counseling programs, and national or local networks of women in prison.

## CURRICULUM DESIGN AND MODES OF DELIVERY

When designing curricula, it is important to consider the mode of delivery as well as the course content. Students' values, attitudes and beliefs need to be considered when deciding which learning activities to employ. Biggs' model of constructive alignment may be referred to when deciding which learning activities will best support the achievement of the intended learning outcomes by each group of participants.[3] Chosen learning activities must take into account participants' learning styles and previous learning experiences in order to promote the engagement of the participant with the content of the curriculum and thus construct learning in line with the intended learning outcomes. The Kolb experiential learning cycle[4] may be used to consider how experience and critical reflection on experience can enable the participant to develop new concepts to guide future practice. The experiential cycle is a four-stage process that moves in sequence through concrete experience, reflection upon experience, and learning from experience to planning and putting into practice/experimenting with what has been learned. This is consistent with the Freire approach with learning through experience leading to transformation and, therefore, consideration needs to be given to how reflection and experiential learning methods can be included within curricula.

It cannot be expected that participants will share the values, beliefs and attitudes of each other or of the facilitator of the teaching and learning experience. An exercise such as values clarification might be helpful in developing awareness of the values both of the participants and the facilitator, and therefore assist in ensuring the course meets some of the needs of the participants. This will also enable the commencement of a reflective process. For many participants reflecting on their previous practice and beliefs might be a difficult process, particularly as they might identify as being part of an oppressed/oppressive group. Therefore the learning environment must be safe for them to be able to be honest and open. Issues identified during the process of reflection might be used as a focus for action learning sets. Action learning sets might be employed for the participant to investigate practices or instigate change in their working environment.

Provision for the development of ongoing support and supervision for participants working in oppressive regimes must be included. They might have been able to reframe their experiences of working in prisons and with prisoners. There must be consideration of the impact for them of returning to work in an oppressive regime when their ideas have been changed by their experiences of teaching, learning and open exchange. While peer support and education are fundamental for the development of prisoners, they are equally important for those working within or around the system. Thus, the experience of undertaking the course could lead to the development of peer support groups. It could be very useful to invite selected prisoners/ex-prisoners to mentor participants in their learning and for them to be involved in assessment of participants' class performance.

### Discussion Topics for Small-Group Work

Below are some of the topics that have been found useful in classes of this kind.

➤ The Russian writer, Fydor Dostoevsky, once said that the best way to understand a society is to visit its prisons. What do you think of this statement? What might a visit to a prison tell us about our society? How does our criminal justice system reinforce existing inequalities of race, class and gender? How do differences of race, class, immigrant status, gender and age affect people's experience with the criminal justice system?

➤ Why has the number of women in prison soared in the last 20–30 years?

➤ What are some of the myths about crime? How do we define crime? Has it changed over time?

➤ How does the prison system touch all of our lives?

➤ What happens when someone goes to jail? How does it affect the individual, the family, the community?

➤ How do the conditions of confinement in penal settings shape individual health?

➤ How does an institution that is supposed to be about public safety become so damaging to our communities?

➤ Why is women's health in prison a public health concern? How is it related to other public health concerns, like the need for drug treatment, violence prevention, etc.?

➤ Are there alternative ways to achieve public safety?

➤ What happens to the children and caregivers left behind when a parent goes to prison? How does this affect the whole community?

➤ Are there other times in history when large numbers of children from an oppressed community have been separated from their parents? Why is this part of social control? What can we do to challenge this?

➤ What role do you see for community health workers in assisting prisoners and their families in the reentry process?

### Experiential Learning Activities

It is important to consider safety, the use of ground rules and ice-breakers when facilitating experiential learning activities. Agreeing on ground rules may give the group greater cohesion, purpose and direction and thus help individual participants to feel that that it is safe to become involved in an open discussion forum. Ice-breakers may also help participants to relax and hopefully be less inhibited when participating in discussion groups.

Role plays may be used to promote experiential learning. However, role plays must be carefully planned with safety, debriefing and an analysis of the role play included within the lesson plan. Examples of experiential learning activities may be found in *Changing Paths: a literacy and life skills program for women in conflict with the law* which has been devised by the Elizabeth Fry Society of Edmonton, Canada.[5]

Enquiry Based Learning (EBL) and Problem Based Learning (PBL) provide opportunities for participants to direct their own learning. Consideration may be given to participants generating their own problem to make the learning activity more "real" and thus promote deep learning.[6]

### Action Learning Sets

Action learning sets (small groups of approximately six people) is a method of teaching and learning that might be employed to help embed learning in the workplace, through enabling participants to explore and potentially address a real problem that they have identified as arising from their practice. Each learning set is encouraged to produce an innovative action plan of work to continue with after the training course has ended. Therefore, the use of action learning sets promotes experiential learning with reflection on practice being moved through to action, thus change within the workplace is promoted. Team working is also encouraged with participants working together outside of the classroom setting and incorporating learning activities into their current and future work.

## SUMMARY

The social justice approach we have adopted in this chapter has explicitly discussed inequities experienced by women incarcerated within criminal justice systems. Highlighted have been issues relating to gender, "race," economic status, education, connectedness to a community and physical and mental health. These demonstrate how a whole range of inequities can result. Teaching and learning about these matters will not directly affect these inequities. However, it can make problematic and raise questions about some of the attitudes and beliefs that may have been simply accepted, not thought about, and taken for granted by those involved in the education process. We do not know whether this will lead to changed ways of thinking about these issues, let alone action directed toward social justice. However, we can live with hope as the vital organizing principle in our lives and belief that change is possible.

## ACKNOWLEDGEMENT

The authors thank Tim Berthold from City College of San Francisco for his support. He approved the curriculum that was developed by Donna Willmott for the course *Incarceration and Health*. He also gave the authors permission to use the curriculum in this chapter. Donna Willmott has taught this course multiple times and continues to revise it.

## REFERENCES

1 Freire P. *Pedagogy of the Oppressed*, translated by Myra Bergman Ramos. New York, NY: Continuum Publishing Company; 1998/1970.
2 Simpson A, Reynolds L, Light I, *et al*. Talking with the experts: evaluation of an online discussion forum involving mental health service users in the education of mental health nursing students. *Nurse Educ Today*. 2008; **28**(5): 633–40.
3 Biggs J. *Teaching for Quality Learning at University*. Buckingham: SRHE and Open University Press; 1999.
4 Kolb D. *Experiential Learning*. Englewood Cliffs, NJ: Prentice Hall; 1984.
5 Sochatsky B, Stewart S. *Changing Paths: a literacy and life skills program for women in conflict with the law*. Edmonton, AB; Elizabeth Fry Society of Edmonton; 2003. Available at: www.nald.ca/clr/changing/changing.pdf (accessed February 28, 2009).
6 Light G, Cox R. *Learning and Teaching in Higher Education*. London: Sage Publications; 2001.

# CHAPTER 13

# Women Prisoners and Health Justice: Challenges and Recommendations

Anastasia Fisher, Diane Hatton and Jane Dorotik

Using a multinational approach with contributors of varying viewpoints, this edited volume takes a broad perspective on issues of relevance to the health of women prisoners in four countries. Advocates, criminologists, current and former prisoners, lawyers, nurses, physicians, and sociologists from Australia, Canada, the UK and US analyze the impact of imprisonment on the physical, mental, and social health of women and their families. In recognizing the unprecedented increase in the number of women prisoners in these four countries, the authors acknowledge the devastating impact of women's imprisonment not only on their well-being but also on their communities, families, and particularly their children. The role of race, class and gender in health, policing and sentencing practices, the environment of prison, and barriers to community reentry is examined throughout. While authors approach their chapter from their own unique perspective, all support a human rights framework for examining how imprisonment further complicates the health disparities of women prisoners. They advocate for limited use of prisons, and social reforms that support rebuilding communities now most heavily affected by mass incarceration policies. It is easy to become overwhelmed by the scope and complexity of the problems; yet, the authors present strategies for improving conditions, changing attitudes and policies, and developing alternatives to incarceration. They recognize that work to change current practices and policies requires leadership, new partnerships, and new ways of thinking about the problems.

This group of authors represents a model of the new partnerships needed to change current practices and policies, and embodies the values of the editors whose journey with this project began with an application to the Rockefeller

Foundation and a belief that an international coalition of advocates, former prisoners, professionals, and social scientists committed to making changes in the lives of women prisoners could make a difference. This book represents a beginning rather than an end; we hope it contributes to dialogue and actions that improve conditions for women prisoners, their families, and their communities and that someday the harms being done in the name of justice are eliminated.

By taking a health justice perspective, the editors of this volume hold the ideal that health for all people is a possibility that requires societies around the world to address inequities, discrimination, and the paralyzing effects of poverty. We find it shameful that inadequate prison health care, in combination with the already poor health prisoners bring into prisons, "results in a pattern of health problems not seen in any other institutional population in the US."[1] This is one reason why we suggest that eliminating the disparities between prison health and public health may not go far enough. Drucker[1] notes that prisoners do not represent a distinct population, but instead are the same people who inhabit the poor and minority communities of the US, and many other nations. The risks and disparities in health care that are the norm in prisons mirror those to which they are exposed in their home community. Additionally, many of the specific health risks and patterns of social injustice faced by prisoners persist after their release. From this description, it is clear that problems of prison health are problems of society and we are reminded of one of the world's most famous former prisoners, Nelson Mandela, who said "no one truly knows a nation until one has been inside its jails. A nation should be judged not by how it treats its highest citizens, but its lowest ones."[2]

## RECOMMENDATIONS FOR ACTION

We close this volume with specific recommendations for actions aimed at improving the health and lives of women prisoners, their families, and communities. Many of these recommendations have been presented by the authors in this volume; others have been identified elsewhere. They are approaches useful for advocates, educators, health professionals, policy makers, prison officials, and members of the public concerned about the health of women prisoners and their communities; they recognize that prison health care cannot be separated from the wider consideration of the nature of imprisonment and its use.[3] Although ambitious, they are available and achievable if we have the will.

1 Use jails and prisons sparingly, especially for non-violent offenses, and replace incarceration with community alternatives such as drug, mental health, and homeless courts, as well as other community-based options.
2 Develop alliances with those who advocate for alternatives to incarceration

and identify pathways by which prison and jail policies damage health.[4]

3 Improve prison health care and programs and integrate them into mainstream public health services.

4 Implement gender-responsive strategies and programs that meet the needs of women prisoners such as those proposed by Bloom, Owen, Covington, and Raeder.[5]

5 Implement standards of, and accreditation for, prison health care.

6 Integrate human rights values and ethics into codes of conduct for prison health care professionals.

7 Develop collaborative partnerships to advocate for the rights of prisoners and those released to the community, including advocating for social reforms that reinvest in low-income communities to reduce recidivism.

8 End discriminatory policies that limit the voting rights, employment opportunities, housing, health and social benefits, and family reunification for persons with felony convictions.

9 Develop and implement curricula for professionals, policy makers, community workers, and members of the public that challenge negative stereotypical ways of thinking about women prisoners and illuminate the socio-political and structural conditions behind incarceration.

10 Repeal mandatory sentencing laws and other criminal justice approaches to social problems, such as homelessness and mental illness, and the "war on drugs."

11 Support and fund the conduct of ethical research involving prisoners.[6]

As in any project of this magnitude, the work will be incomplete and gaps will remain. Those of us committed to this work are faced with horrific problems and significant challenges. California, the home state of the editors, provides an example of the problems and challenges found in prison health care. Judge Henderson, in his 2005 decision to establish a receivership taking control of the delivery of medical services provided to all California state prisoners confined by the California Department of Corrections and Rehabilitation, stated in part:

> By all accounts, the California prison medical care system is broken beyond repair. The harm already done in this case to California's prison inmate population could not be more grave and the threat of future injury and death is virtually guaranteed in the absence of drastic action. It is an uncontested fact that, on average, an inmate in one of California's prisons needlessly dies every six to seven days due to constitutional deficiencies in the CDCR's [California Department of Corrections and Rehabilitation's] medical delivery system. It is clear to the Court that this unconscionable degree of suffering and death is sure to continue if the system is not dramatically overhauled. Decades of neglecting

medical care while vastly expanding the size of the prison system has led to a state of institutional paralysis. The prison system is unable to function effectively and suffers a lack of will with respect to prisoner medical care.[7]

This example provides a cautionary tale to those in other nations. The unprecedented increase in the worldwide prison population is well documented[1,8–10] as are the serious health problems of prisoners.[11–21] If left unaddressed, these conditions can lead to the types of horrors described by Judge Henderson.

To improve the lives of women prisoners requires societies that value women reinvest in their communities and their children, and use prisons only as a last resort for the very few. We have a choice. We can continue to punish people or we can tackle the problems of inequity, discrimination and the paralyzing effects of poverty, and work to achieve health justice.

## REFERENCES

1 Drucker EM. Incarcerated people. In: Levy BS, Sidel VW, editors. *Social Injustice and Public Health*. Oxford: Oxford University Press; 2006. pp. 161–75.

2 Mandela N. *Long Walk to Freedom: the autobiography of Nelson Mandela*. Boston: Back Bay Books; 1995.

3 Coyle A. Conclusion. In: Coyle A, Campbell A, Neufeld R, editors. *Capitalist Punishment: prison privatization and human rights*. Atlanta, GA: Clarity Press; 2003. pp. 211–18.

4 Freudenberg N. Adverse effects of US jail and prison policies on the health and well-being of women of color. *Am J Public Health*. 2002; 92(12): 1895–9.

5 Bloom B, Owen B, Covington S, *et al. Gender-Responsive Strategies: research, practice, and guiding principles for women offenders*. Washington, DC: National Institute of Corrections; 2003. Available at: www.nicic.org/pubs/2003/018017.pdf (accessed February 17, 2009).

6 Institute of Medicine. *Ethical Considerations for Research Involving Prisoners*. Washington, DC: The National Academies Press; 2007.

7 Henderson TE. Findings of Fact and Conclusions of Law Re: Appointment of Receiver, Marciano Plata, *et al.* vs Arnold Schwarzenegger, *et al.* US District Court of the Northern District of California; October 3, 2005. p. 2. Available at: www.cprinc.org/docs/court/PlataFindingsFactConclusionsLaw1005.pdf (accessed May 25, 2009).

8 Sudbury J, editor. *Global Lockdown: race, gender, and the prison-industrial complex*. New York, NY: Routledge; 2005.

9 Walmsley R. Prison planet. *Foreign Policy*. 2007; 160(May/Jun): 30–1.

10 Wood PJ. The rise of the prison industrial complex in the United States. In: Coyle A, Campbell A, Neufeld R, editors. *Capitalist Punishment: prison privatization and human rights*. Atlanta, GA: Clarity Press; 2003. pp. 16–29.

11 Braithwaite RL, Arriola KJ, Newkirk C. *Health Issues Among Incarcerated Women*. New Brunswick, NJ: Rutgers University Press; 2006.

12 Braithwaite RL, Treadwell HM, Arriola KR. Health disparities and incarcerated women: a population ignored. *Am J Public Health*. 2005; 95(10): 1679–81.

13 Fogel CI, Belyea M. Psychological risk factors in pregnant inmates: a challenge for nursing. *MCN Am J Matern Child Nurs.* 2001; **26**(1): 10–16.

14 Freudenberg N, Daniels J, Crum M, *et al.* Coming home from jail: the social and health consequences of community reentry for women, male adolescents, and their families and communities. *Am J Public Health.* 2005; **95**(10): 1725–36.

15 Freudenberg N, Moseley J, Labriola M, *et al.* Comparison of health and social characteristics of people leaving New York City jails by age, gender, and race/ethnicity: implications for public health interventions. *Public Health Reports.* 2007; **122**(6): 733–43.

16 Hatton DC, Kleffel D, Fisher AA. Prisoners' perspectives of health problems and healthcare in a US women's jail. *Women and Health.* 2006; **44**(1): 119–36.

17 National Commission on Correctional Health Care. *The Health Status of Soon-To-Be-Released Inmates: a report to Congress.* Available at: www.ncchc.org/pubs/pubs_stbr.html (accessed February 28, 2009).

18 Pratt D, Piper M, Appleby L, *et al.* Suicide in recently released prisoners: a population-based cohort study. *Lancet.* 2006; **368**(9530): 119–23.

19 Stoller N. *Improving Access to Health Care for California's Women Prisoners.* Berkeley, CA: California Policy Research Center, University of California; 2001. Available at: http://cpac.berkeley.edu/documents/stollerpaper.pdf (accessed May 24, 2009).

20 Stoller N. Space, place and movement as aspects of health care in three women's prisons. *Soc Sci Med.* 2003; **56**(11): 2263–75.

21 Willmott D, van Olphen J. Challenging the health impacts of incarceration: the role for community health workers. *Californian J Health Promot.* 2005; **3**(2): 38–48.

# Index